THE CARDS WE'RE DEALT

And the Joker is Lupus

By:

Marilyn Celeste Morris

Dedication:

To all who struggle daily with the disease of Systemic Lupus
Erythematosus
And
To the memory of all who have lost their struggle with The Wolf

Acknowledgements:

To the Lupies Yahoo group, individually and together, for their contributions, using their collective wisdom, their unique talents of expressing themselves, their humor and all-encompassing love for each other.

Special thanks to Sandra, Grandma Barb and Mary Mike, owners of the list, for granting me the privilege of quoting messages from the board.

To those who contributed from other Lupus support sites;

To the Lupus Foundation of America, for providing information about this puzzling illness, and sponsoring the many fund raising events both locally and nationally.

Foreword

In 1988, I began journaling about my strange symptoms, my frustrations and anger as I sought diagnosis and treatment of what would eventually be diagnosed as Systemic Lupus Erythematosus (Lupus.) I later realized I could incorporate many of the entries into a book, which was published in 2005 as *Diagnosis: Lupus: The Intimate Journal of a Lupus Patient.*

Since that time, I have learned a great deal from others suffering from this quixotic disease, and I began formulating a plan for this book.

My purpose, as it was with the original publication, is to inform, in non-clinical language, newly-diagnosed, yet-to-be diagnosed patients and their families; give them courage to continue seeking a diagnosis in the face of frustration and feelings of despair; and offer hope, even when conditions seem hopeless.

By relating our innermost thoughts and feelings, I hope readers will come to realize they are not alone in their frustration, depression, job losses and subsequent loss of income, battles with an alphabet soup of public assistance services, Social Security Disability and food stamps.

Questions such as "How did I get this disease? Will my children also get it? Why doesn't my doctor tell me anything except "You've got Lupus; take this medicine and come back in three months" will be addressed, along with many others.

Although many journal entries detail my struggles with clinical depression, job losses, loss of income and other dire consequences of this disease, my intent is not to linger there, but to press on toward acceptance, remission, and recovery.

As many new members of a Lupus Support Group sigh in relief upon finding us, "I thought I was the only person in the world who felt this way," so will readers discover they are truly not alone in their thinking and their feelings.

While I compiled these entries from the perspective of a "recovering" Lupus patient, I was also aware that Lupus might rear its ugly head at any moment, bringing me back to the rounds of physicians, medications, and even hospitalization. This is the life anyone with any chronic disease must lead, and their choices are either to feel sorry for themselves and burrow into a sinkhole of despair, or live life as it comes, one day at a time, the best way possible.

I have known persons who have lost the battle and I certainly want to live a long and healthy life.

I also know that tomorrow, my life may be ended in a freak accident.

My decision is, "I'm not going to stop living just so I can live."

Introduction

May 2002

"Are you sure you have Lupus?" My newest doctor asked as he entered the exam room, my lab tests from the week before in his hands.

"Yes. I was diagnosed in Oct. 1988," I replied. "Why? What do the tests show?"

"Well, they show no sign of Lupus. Sed rate is normal, no RA factor…"

"Great!" I burbled. "Suppose I'm in remission?"

"Or maybe you never really had Lupus." He shrugged.

For one crazy, hopeful moment, I actually thought: "Maybe he's right. Maybe I didn't really have Lupus, after all."

Then my thoughts flooded to the three years of constant joint pain, lab tests, five doctors telling me it was either "all in my head" or "Just rheumatoid arthritis" all the while being told not enough symptoms were showing in the blood work.

Never really had Lupus?_ I wanted to shout: Then what was all the lung infection, the hair loss, the treatments with Cytoxan, Imuran, prednisone; the difficulty walking when vasculitis caused foot drop in both feet and I fell down a lot? Frustration mounted on frustration as the disease progressed.

Never really had Lupus? Then what was with my red, swollen joints, causing one rheumatologist to rhapsodise, "What beautiful swollen knees!" When I couldn't wear rings, watches or bracelets because of the intense pain and swelling? When even my collarbones hurt?

Never really had Lupus? Then what was all the bouncing from job to job, being fired or quitting due to sheer physical exhaustion, or finding it impossible to concentrate on the task at hand?

Never really had Lupus? Then why did I break out in a fiery rash after being in the sun? What was the point in hauling my body out of bed at 5:30 a.m., climbing painfully into a tub of hot water, eating breakfast so I could swallow my handful of meds (that didn't seem to be doing much good) so I could get dressed and have my butt in a chair at my office-du-jour by 8:00 a.m.?

Never really had Lupus? Then what was all the memory loss about? What words escaped me at just the right time to embarrass me so that I could only shrug and murmur, "Lupus lapse."

Rather than lash out at this newest, most optimistic young doctor, I merely smiled and shrugged, "Yes, I really did, and I really do have Lupus."

I wish I could tell you that my disease came on suddenly, that I went to the doctor, was diagnosed and treated immediately, and everybody lived happily ever after.

Unfortunately, that didn't happen. Nor does it happen with the majority of Lupus patients; at least with those I've known. After three years full of pain, doubt, fear, and anger, and after changing doctors, both primary care physicians and rheumatologists, *five* times, I was at last diagnosed with SLE.

And my treatment took a very long time, and brought with it, not the expected relief of pain, doubt, fear and anger, but *Four (Other) Horsemen of This Disease*: Weight gain, high blood pressure, diabetes, and vasculitis. I must also add clinical depression, job loss, loss of income, foreclosure, lining up for food stamps, medicines and other Public Assistance services. I was truly humbled when I picked up my handicapped parking tag, food stamps and vouchers.

I was infuriated by low-level clerks who used their positions of power to assert their superiority over me, verbally slapping my wrists, and at one point, one even shaking her finger at me, yet I had to submit in order to get whatever assistance they could offer.

I had a meltdown in my parish priest's office, confessing that I needed financial help; I had a true gasping-for-air, snot-slinging hissy fit in the college library when I was told I might not be able to complete my schooling. And all this time, I tried to reassure my family and friends that I would not, could not, leave this crappy world via my own hand, even though I admitted, however, I **would** like to just **lie down and die**.

That's what this disease did *to* me.

* * * *

This is what this disease did *for* me.

I learned there is a God, and I'm not Him/Her.

I learned that God loves me as much as he loves you.

I learned I'm not perfect, never have been, never will be, and that's okay.

I learned that this disease is not a punishment for "sins."

I learned how to ask for help.

I learned how to be grateful for and accept that help.

I learned that things are merely objects, that money is simply a means to an end, and not the be-all and end-all of life.

I learned the difference between *needs* and *wants.*

I learned to surrender, to "Let go and let God."

I learned that expectations are only pre-meditated resentments.

I learned not to discount the message because of the messenger.

If any of the above sounds vaguely familiar to those of you who are members of a 12-Step Recovery group, you are correct. I make no secret of the fact that I am a grateful member of the Al-Anon Family Group, and lest anyone fear I am breaking my anonymity, my last name is not the same as my children's or my ex-husband's, since I wisely had my maiden name restored upon my divorce.

When I mention friends' names, some are members of the fellowship, some are not. I have, however, changed the names of the doctors and institutions, simply because I believe it serves no purpose to impugn their reputations. I also know today that they did the best they could with the information available at the time. They're not perfect, and they certainly aren't gods.

When I write of my parents' shortcomings, I am not "parent-bashing" or playing "Let's blame Mom and Dad." My parents weren't perfect, any more than my doctors were perfect; they also did the best they could in trying to cope with their feelings about my illness.

I give thanks daily that I was already a member of the Al-Anon Family Group and the Episcopal Church before the onset of symptoms of SLE. While working with my sponsor, while studying to be a Stephen Minister, and while literally crying on my dear friends' shoulders, I was sustained by their love and caring support. By holding me in their arms, keeping me in their prayers, and yes, by giving me swift kicks to the posterior when I needed it, these people kept me alive.

To this day, I don't know how they managed to listen to my constant crying, complaints, and self-doubts, much less stand by stoically as they heard me rage at God, myself and the entire universe for whatever was going wrong in my life.

Because of them, I am alive. Today.

And I know today that is all we have – This day. This moment.

I hope my experiences inform you, strengthen you, and give you hope.

First, Some Facts...

Some symptoms of Lupus:

Do you have/ever had/been told you have:

Achy, painful and/or swollen joints for more than three months;

Fingers and/or toes becoming pale, numb or uncomfortable in the cold;

Sores in the mouth for more than two weeks;

Been told you have a low blood count, anemia, low white cell count or a low platelet count;

Ever had a prominent redness or color change in the shape of a butterfly across the bridge of your nose and cheeks;

An unexplained fever over 100 degrees for more than a few days;

A sensitivity to the sun where the skin breaks out after being in the sun (not a sunburn);

Had chest pain with breathing for more than a few days (pleurisy);

Been told you had protein in your urine;

Experienced persistent, extreme fatigue and weakness for days or weeks at a time even after 6-8 hours of restful nighttime sleep.

If you have 3 or more symptoms, you should see your doctor.

According to the Lupus Foundation of America, Lupus is more common than Leukemia, Hodgkin's Disease, Muscular Dystrophy, Cystic Fibrosis and Multiple Sclerosis. And yet, the average person rarely knows about Lupus and is generally misinformed, vaguely believing it to be "kind of like arthritis, isn't it?" While my symptoms first presented themselves as "kind of like arthritis," and I was thus diagnosed and treated for two years for RA, other symptoms soon presented themselves, until, after three emotionally charged and pain-filled years from the onset of symptoms, laboratory tests confirmed the presence of SLE, or Systemic Lupus Erythematosus.

There are two distinct types of Lupus. One is discoid Lupus, where the skin shows large "splotches" or red rashes in clusters, mostly on the face, across the cheeks and the bridge of the nose, creating a "wolf-like" mask. One can have discoid Lupus and systemic Lupus at the same time; generally, those who suffer with the discoid form of Lupus do not develop the systemic form. But, in keeping with the nature of this beast, sometimes they do.

The second is systemic Lupus; that is, it is throughout the body. It has been classified as "an autoimmune disease."

Lupus has nothing to do with AIDS, I must point out. With AIDS, the immune system is destroyed. With Lupus, the immune system is on overdrive. I like the 'short', understandable description of what Lupus is: Think of the body as a fort, like in the Wild West Days. Every now and then, Indians attack the fort, and the soldiers inside the fort (immune system) repel the Indians (the infection). Then the fort (body) settles down and goes back to its usual routine, until the next Indian attack

But with Lupus, there are no Indians. The soldiers inside the fort are ever ready for an attack, but the Indians don't arrive, so the soldiers (stressed) turn on each other, fighting among themselves, eventually destroying the fort itself: lungs, kidneys, central nervous system, and other vital organs.

As of this printing, there is no cure, but it is treatable.

Words to the Newly Diagnosed, Undiagnosed and Their Families....

Actually, one word. Hope. There *is* hope. Despite the pain, the despair, the uncertainty, and the fatigue – there is a light at the end of the tunnel. While listening to new members of our local Lupus support group, I hear their fear.

"I thought I was the only person in the world who felt this way."

"Did your doctor tell you it was all in your head?"

"Did your doctor tell you it was 'just' rheumatoid arthritis?"

"My family does not understand what I'm going through. After all, I don't look sick."

"How can you work when you have Lupus?"

"How can I get social security disability? They keep denying my claim."

"My company fired me after I took disability. Is this legal?"

"How can I find work when I'm so sick?"

"How do you manage the pain?"

"What does cortisone do to your body?"

"Why isn't the medication my doctor prescribed for me doing me any good? I still hurt."

"Why doesn't my doctor tell me more about Lupus? All he said was, 'You have Lupus. Take this medicine and come back in three months.'"

"My doctor won't talk to me when I call his office. His office staff tells me he's busy, or he can't talk to me, and they won't answer my questions. What should I do?"

"How do I answer people's questions when I tell them I have Lupus?"

And, the topper: "People tell me 'You don't look sick. You look too healthy to be sick.'"

And their unspoken questions, as much as those uttered: "Will I die from this? How long will I be sick? Will I get worse? What about kidney involvement? Seizures? Why did I get this disease? Will my children also get it"?

Difficult questions, indeed.

I must address the disgraceful ideas espoused by the ignorant that that you must have not lived a good, clean life, or you wouldn't have developed cancer, diabetes, --- or SLE. If only you hadn't taken aspartame.... If only. Blame the victim. You don't blame the caner patient, do you?

However, I do believe with the perception that stress plays a major role in illness' development, and, Lord knows, I had enough stress in my life.

And so does everyone

Stress, good or bad (marriage, children being born, promotions, are all stressors) has an effect on one's mind and body. By the time I reached age 44, I had had several major stressors, and I reacted the way I always had – chin up, swallowed my hurt and anger, and got on with it.

Most of us Lupies have had a great deal of stress in our lives. We are, after all, over-achievers. We take on more than the ordinary person. We are perfectionists. We work too hard, don't know how to play, and don't rest when we should. And that's *before* we get Lupus. So it's extremely difficult to "take it easy" when diagnosed with this disease.

So with my stress, I didn't take the time to grieve over my divorces, to rage aloud at the injustices in my life.
I simmered. And my body, seeking an outlet for such stress build-up, rebelled. Like volcanoes, fires erupted in my joints, cartilage and ligaments. My emotional pain had been crying out to me.

But it was *physical pain* that got my attention.

What my personal journey through this darkness has taught me is this: The disease is worst at the beginning – before diagnosis and treatment.

As in my case, I was diagnosed in October, 1988 and hospitalized with a raging case of pleuritis in March 1989. This was preceded, of course, by at least three years of constant searching for a diagnosis, going from doctor to doctor, bouncing from job to job as my energy level waned and deteriorated, and dealing with an alphabet soup of medical institutions, insurance companies, mental health and rehabilitation facilities. And then, despite the aggressive treatment, my body succumbed at last

But back to the statement: It's worse in the beginning.

Once the lab tests and your doctor's best guess confirm a positive indicator for SLE, and treatment is begun, you can get better. I promise. You might also get worse before you get better. I promise that, too. But you will get to the point where the pain abates, anxiety lessens, mobility is restored and confidence in living a full life returns.

It will take time, medications, and dedication on your part to adhere to the treatment plan your physician has outlined for you, keeping in mind "You must become your own best physician," and determination to defeat this beast, this wolf, that has taken up residence in your body.

A support system is essential. Family, friends, church – learn to lean on them for a change. I know, we have always been the ones to comfort, rather than be comforted. To give, rather than receive, care, compassion and chicken soup to those in need.

Now it's your turn.

Embarrassed? It's nothing you did or didn't do. It happens. Through no fault of yours, or your ancestry, or you didn't lead a "good life"…

Still, I questioned: "Why me?" "Why now?"

Because, that's why, my mother/myself said.

I did cry a lot when the Lupus was at its worst. I wanted the pain to end; although I didn't want to actually commit suicide, there were times when I sincerely wanted to just lie down and die.

While looking back on my journals for use in writing this book, I was struck by what seemed at first as an inordinate amount of "whining." But, by golly, I needed to whine. Indeed, I not only "whined," I complained. I ranted. Frustrated beyond belief, I lashed out at those around me. And I railed against God Himself.

Yet somehow, I was sustained through this challenging time in my life. I attained an unexpected spiritual growth in the face of this adversity. Years ago, I would have gagged on the "goody two shoes" phrases, believing there was noting "spiritual" about having any illness. God was against me, if He existed at all, and certainly, I didn't feel "noble" about suffering with this dammed disease.

I took heart from one of the many books I read where one of the chapters was titled, *Dying Is the Easy Part*. I knew it would be easier to die than to stand up and fight this disease. I've never been known to take the easy way out.

So I allowed myself to cry.

My doctor said, "You've got a right to sing the blues," and sing them I did.

I had the determination to beat this disease, but I needed help – beyond that of modern medicine.

* * * *

"Life is Difficult" *M. Scott Peck wrote in* The Road Less Traveled.

Nobody had ever told me that before. Any little annoyance, inconvenience, or major lifestyle change caused me to rebel. "It's not fair. Life isn't supposed to be like this. Bad things happen to other people, but not to me. I've been good."

Rabbi Harold Kushner wrote pretty much the same thing in his landmark book: *When Bad Things Happen to Good People* and the truth finally dawned on me: *Life happens*. With or without my permission or approval.

Laughter is essential. Norman Cousins, in his book, *Anatomy of an Illness*, tells how he rented a hotel room, a projector and old Marx Brothers movies, and laughed his way out of the pain. A good 30 minutes of laughter enabled him to sleep where he could not before.

I began keeping a journal. After all, I had whined to my family and friends enough. I needed to vent. I needed to feel sorry for myself even while I presented a brave front to the world. This journal led me to a special kind of healing. I began a physical and spiritual journey, realizing one cannot be undertaken without the other.

I would someday use these entries for my story about Lupus, I thought. But when every other journal entry contained references to laments of financial worries, fear and insecurities, I wondered, "Who would want to wade through all these recitations of woe? Reading about chronic illness is not a favorite choice, anyway; if a person has Lupus. Isn't it enough to just read the facts and go on?"

No, it isn't, in my humble opinion. I could read all the statistics in the world and still not feel like anyone understands how I feel – what's actually going on inside me, emotionally, as well as dry numbers on a sed rate scale. More than anything else, I believe, I wanted people to know that the pain I was experiencing encompassed more than every joint/connective tissue/vital organ of my body. That pain influenced every area of my life...physical, mental, emotional and spiritual.

I wanted people to know that I was, indeed, legitimately suffering from the slings and arrows of outrageous fortune, even though I "looked wonderful."

Because Lupus patients truly don't "look sick." Unlike cancer, Lupus does not leave its victims looking pale, gaunt, and emaciated. We appear in radiant good health, while Lupus may be silently destroying our kidneys. We look – ahem – overfed, overweight – pumped up on steroids, our faces get rounder and rounder; our trunks also bloom while the limbs remain the same. An odd appearance, to say the least, and one that is not welcomed by its hosts, prompting remarks such as "How can you be so sick when you look so – uh – (Say it—dammit! fat!) healthy." Personally, I'd rather be 20 pounds over my ideal weight, walking around, than skinny in my coffin.

We generally have no visible disabilities, either, like Parkinson's patients. There are usually no tremors, no speech difficulties, and no problems with ambulating. Certain forms of Lupus, of course, can lead to seizures, psychoses, and other neurological defects, but generally, we appear healthy.

Treatment for Lupus is non-dramatic, as a cancer's chemotherapy. Yes, we take pills. Lots of pills. Generally, we are not forced into being "hooked up to tubes" intravenously. But the meds also give us hair loss, violent rashes and scars on our fragile skin, and our eyes must be protected from the sunlight.

Many of us work, at least part-time, as our illness allows. Sometimes we go into remission, for days, weeks, months, years, and we rejoice in those times. But when Lupus bites into us, wearing us down with fatigue, pain, arthritic-like hands, swollen knees, mal-functioning kidneys, and neurological misfires, we are truly, once again, very sick.

Even if we still look in the best of health. Some days you're the bug, some days you're the windshield.

My Search Begins

From My Journals

VICTIM: A living being used as a sacrifice in a religious ceremony, a person or thing destroyed or hurt in the pursuit of some object; one injured or killed by some misfortune or calamity; a sufferer from mental or physical disease; a dupe.

SUFFER: To feel (up-bear) what is painful, disagreeable or distressing; endure with pain or distress; as to suffer a wrong; to feel or bear upward, as to suffer pain; to be affected by, exercise, undergo; to allow; permit; To experience pain, loss, distress. Endure, support, tolerate.

I searched for a label to pin on my puzzling symptoms:

The inability to type all day at a computer. The inability to sit, stand and walk for eight hours in a day without extreme fatigue. The inability to understand and implement simple verbal instructions due to a puzzling and devastating "fog" that enveloped my cognitive functions at crucial moments. And, if it hadn't been so critical to my job performance, the temporary loss of verbal ability resulting in garbled and stuttering answers to my supervisors' questions. Needless to say, I was "let go" several times.

Some diseases begin so dramatically, so definitively, that there is no question in any physician's mind as to the diagnosis. A lump in the breast calls for immediate biopsy and lab tests. A sudden sharp pain in the chest sends the patient to the emergency room where high-tech equipment confirms the presence of heart disease.

Not so with Lupus. This disease presents itself with such a myriad of symptoms that its sufferers doubt their sanity. Pain, stiffness in the joints surely must mean arthritis-- or, as several of my former physicians dismissed it casually, "After all, at your age, just learn to live with it."

Sudden and dramatic weight loss, a boon to any woman struggling with her self-image ("Well, I see you've lost a lot of weight recently. Good for you; keep it up.") Instead of an alarm that something is wrong. Other symptoms, such as extreme fatigue cause even the patient to question herself. "Tired? How can I be so tired that I just want to lie down and not even move? I must be lazy. No, I really have to nap before dinner.... *what is wrong with me?*"

Weeks, even months pass, with no improvement. Symptoms worsen. After the family physician, his knowledge exhausted, extensive lab tests reveal nothing unusual, the patient is labeled a hypochondriac. There is *really nothing wrong,* she is told.

But the pain makes believing this difficult. While seated on a stool in the shower, unable to stand, the woman notices in horror that large clumps of hair are flowing down the drain. When she manages to pull herself together for some social event, she teeters on the brink of exhaustion only to be scolded on the way home by her husband/companion/family:

"I don't understand how you can be so tired all the time. The doctor says there's nothing wrong, with all the expensive lab tests...." leaving the rest of the sentence unspoken. "It's all in your head."

After a time, after months and years of unrelenting, unforgiving, baffling, excruciating, agonizing, subtle, intense, bouts of fatigue and other odd symptoms. Resignation sets in. If relationships are good to begin with, the family considers the patient somewhat "strange," and tolerates her odd behavior pattern with dark humor, somewhat like keeping a crazy maiden aunt locked in the attic. Already strained marriages or other relationships, on the other hand, crack wide open and the partner's psychosomatic "illnesses" provide a good excuse for leaving the marriage or severing the relationship.

Even within the community of family or friends, an undiagnosed Lupus patient is left to cope as best she can --— feeling useless, burdensome to others, sometimes to the point of suicide.

After all, nobody can believe that this person who shows no obvious physical signs of disease,is indeed, ill. In fact, she is 'glowing with good health," apparently, and gaining weight, to boot. The weight gain, moon face, trunk swollen with an extra twenty or thirty pounds, on average comes after massive doses of Prednisone quells the initial pain of the disease but the toll it takes on one's body, and emotions, begins to show.

A young woman who had been a model in her pre-Lupus days, gains one hundred pounds, breaks a hip through necrosis, loses her marvelous long black hair, can't find work due to the pain involved in simple movements, moves back to her parents house, and she becomes suicidal.

There is nothing left before her except more pain, more days full of idleness, seeing her swollen body day after day negating the happy, vivacious creature she was a few short months earlier.

I was a little older than the typical Lupus patient, but I fit the other profile. Lupus patients (or, Lupies) are busy people, working and playing 25 hours a day. They don't know when to quit; they are perfectionists and they have an unquenchable interest in nearly everything.

Their pain threshold is astonishing; I was typical in the way I ignored the first symptoms until they became almost unbearable. Likewise, the tolerance for stress. My motto was, "What stress?" and I was really quite unaware of the tremendous amounts of stress I had been under during most of my life, particularly the last few years.

When I told people that I had Lupus, I got one of several reactions: "What's that?" or, "Lupus? Don't people die from that?" "Do you throw fits or something?" One callous person even asked, "Is it fatal?" and I shot back with, "Life is fatal. "

Bless my friends' hearts; they understood when I had to cancel a social event at the last minute, because I was "crashing" where I had been "fine" a few moments earlier.

How did this disease come to reside in me?

Heredity had a large part in my illness: My mother's mother, Emily Richardson, was half Native American; my mother was born in Sels, Arizona and spent the first three years of her life on the Indian Reservation there. On my father's side, I claim a great-great grandmother, Pernicia Blackwell, who had some Seminole Indian background. (Native American Indians and African-Americans are prime targets of Lupus.)

Besides the ordinary childhood diseases, chickenpox at age 6, mumps at the age of 12, and chronic bronchitis until I "outgrew it" at age 14, I contracted diphtheria in infancy. One of my first memories – if not my very first memory, is of lying on a bed with warm steam rising to the top of a makeshift "tent" of sheets as I struggled for every breath.

This memory surfaced dramatically and unexpectedly when at the ripe old age of 60, I arrived at the emergency room one evening suffering full-blown asthma and the well-meaning nurse thrust a steaming mask at my face; I shot up off the gurney in a visceral, knee-jerk reaction, striking at her hand in an infantile way. She backed off while I sat, perplexed at my response, and then she offered me a mouth tube, which I gladly accepted.

A few weeks after a hysterectomy, I felt absolutely wonderful, invigorated, euphoric, and didn't need any sleep, thank you very much. I ate ravenously, yet lost weight. Finally, after noticing my hands shook all the time, I was convinced that maybe I should pay a visit to the family doctor.

"Are you taking speed?" he asked bluntly.

"Of course not," I huffed.

"Well, you're almost ready to stroke out. I'm sending you to a specialist. Right away."

The specialist determined I had hyperthyroidism and sent me to a radiologist, whereby after drinking a radium cocktail, my thyroid was dissolved. We took off to Aspen CO for a few weeks vacation, where all I could manage to do was sleep; I didn't want to eat, *couldn't* eat, yet I returned home ten pounds heavier. Then it was time to begin thyroid replacement therapy.

This marriage limped along until 1982, and although I mourned the loss of another marriage, I was much too busy to grieve properly.

I began feeling some fatigue, so tired I could hardly get out of bed. I returned to the specialist who had treated my hyperthyroidism, and he suggested I might have a hormone imbalance. "Why don't you try taking Provera?" he suggested, writing out the prescription, which I dutifully had filled.

A bell should have gone off in my head, if not my doctor's. Since it is believed that an excess of hormones can trigger Lupus, and this was the third hormone that my body was now being asked to process, I believe it was too much. It was totally unnecessary for me to have taken that drug. But at the time, I didn't question my doctor.

I do now.

Two months later, my symptoms began...

I woke up with my fingers so swollen I couldn't make my morning pot of coffee. I visited my family doctor, who pronounced, "Looks like arthritis." He prescribed an anti-inflammatory, which didn't work.

I then noticed a vague aching in arms, as if I had carried heavy books all day.

Wrists became involved next; nieces playing with my watch and bracelet was excruciating. Extreme fatigue and weight loss. Rash on "V" neck, fiery red as though I had been in the sun a very long time.

My Primary Care Physician was at a loss. "Probably just arthritis. After all, at your age..." *Thanks a lot for reminding me,* I thought.

The intensity of my physical pain increased to the point that nothing was alleviating it.

By now, I was working for a sole practitioner attorney, who specialized in workers' compensation and personal injury. I was struggling with the incredible fatigue, joint pain and swelling. Incredible pain, all over my body. My wrists were on fire, my knees swollen to the size of grapefruit. And nothing helped. Not aspirin, Advil, hot baths. Nothing.

My office moved to a building under construction. While workers were literally building around me all day long, I breathed fumes from paints, lacquers, varnish and carpet glue, not to mention cringing at the ear-splitting screams of sheet metal being cut and drills boring into concrete.

I again went to my primary care physician who prescribed Feldene and told me to come back if I didn't get better.

I didn't.

I need to see somebody who knows what's going on, I thought. I asked a friend of a friend who was the wife of a physician. She ought to know.

"Dr. Charles Smith" (the true identity of all doctors in this narrative have been changed) she suggested. "He's expensive, but he's good."

I didn't care, at this point, now, with my knees being a prime target. I would see him at any price.

After an extensive examination, Dr. Smith intoned, "It is my considered opinion that you have Lupus. I have no proof, so we will have to run some lab tests. In the meantime," he said, writing out the first of many prescriptions, "no more Naprocin. We'll use an anti-malarial drug that works well on Lupus. It will take three months for it to begin working," he said, "but the pain will be lessened."

"Okay, great!"

"But there are some side effects," he cautioned.

"What side effects?"

"It affects the eyes. Your vision could be affected."

"You mean, as in blind? I could go blind?"

"I need for you to have a visual field base checkup, and then you must have your eyes examined every six months."

As I paid his exorbitant bill, I pondered this new medication and its effects, filled the prescription at my friendly neighborhood pharmacy (the pharmacist and I would become very good friends through the years) and went back to the office, where our clerk was anxiously awaiting my diagnosis.

"Well," I began, "There's good news and there's bad news. The good news is, this new medicine should take effect in about three months and then the pain will be gone. The bad news is, this same medicine might cause me to go blind.

"Some choice," I wailed. "I can either hurt or go blind."

No diagnosis, no relief from my pain, so I was out of there.

One night, I was overcome with pain, and my throat was "closing up." I couldn't breathe well. I called a friend, and told her I was about to die.

She rushed me to the emergency room, where I demanded a cortisone shot. I knew they worked, short term, from previous experiments by my various doctors. I made myself obnoxious by shouting "I probably have Lupus and I need a cortisone shot. *Now*."

I congratulated myself on my assertiveness (actually I was downright hostile.) I was beginning to treat myself, as I had been told in the very beginning of seeking a diagnosis.

"If it is Lupus, it will be a "Do-I-Yourself" disease. *You* must chart your *own* recovery."

My friend took me home where I slept, pain—free, for the remainder of the night.

As I took the medication for the third month, and my pain had not been lessened, I was true to my word…I was Out of There.

Other Various Therapies, Treatments: Reflexology, Biofeedback, Visual Therapy –

I attended a workshop on visual therapy – I was urged to let the child in me draw and paint, willy-nilly, then to draw how I would conquer my disease

I drew an angel with a large golden sword, who touched me on various places of my body, sending a brilliant golden light searing through the cells, infusing them with holy light. I am kneeling in front of the angel. My guardian angel.

Shortly after this course ended, I was strolling in the mall with my boyfriend du jour when I spotted a print I had had as a small child over my bed at my grandmother's house. I'm sure everyone is familiar with it: A guardian angel guides two small children across a wooden bridge, over a raging stream, while lightning flashes in the background. Of course, I bought it.

When I mentioned this to an aunt at a family gathering, she snorted, "Well, I don't know why you think you were so crazy about that painting. When you were a little girl, you were always afraid the bridge would break."

Oh, me of little faith!

I Go to Counselling.

Somewhere, in some dusty archive bin, is a videotape of me sobbing my heart out to a patient Brite Divinity School Graduate. I agreed to the taping because (1) the price of counseling was just right (as I recall, almost free) (2) the location and times were convenient for me and (3) I really had no other choice at the time. We determined (1) that I had felt abandoned as a child, since my father was in the military and he had frequent deployments, (2) I fell into loveless and spiritually abusive relationships; (3) I have a really crappy disease that nobody understands and I'm angry about it. Finally, I was surprised to learn that I am stronger than I thought. All the women in my family history have been strong women. So why not me? I was assured I would survive this crisis.

Doctor #2

I See a Female Physician

"Go see Evelyn Brown," a friend suggested, when I told her my story. "She's a rheumatologist." I thought. "She might understand the pain I'm in, and being a woman, she wouldn't brush it off as psychosomatic."

I hobbled into her office one raw, rainy morning, knees swollen to the point where it was difficult to walk.

"Hop right up here, Ms. Morris," her nurse patted the examination table, high as Mt. Everest to me at that point.

"*Hop?*' I said. "You're asking me to *hop up*?"

She flushed, and then softened. "Here's a step stool; it should be a little easier for you."

She left the room and returned a moment later with the interminable paper work. "Dr. Brown will be in to see you in a few minutes."

I diligently filled in all the blanks while seated on the high examining table, legs dangling (surely this can't do my knees a whole lot of good, I speculated)- and wondering why I had to put on this flimsy paper gown when all that needed to be looked at was my knees. Today, that is, although I still hurt in every joint in my body, today it was the knees that suffered the most.

As I finished the last question on the lengthy paperwork, the door opened and the Renowned Dr. Evelyn Brown entered.

She went straight to the point.

Her point.

"What beautiful swollen knees!" she rhapsodized, poking at them none too gently.

"Do they hurt?"

Do they hurt? I barely restrained myself from yelling out loud. Of course they hurt! I must have said something to that effect, or else she read my leap toward the ceiling as proof enough that yes, I was hurting.

"Hot," she said briskly. "Your joints are hot. Especially first thing in the morning, right? I'll prescribe hot paraffin for you...you could soak your hands in it."

And I was treated to a hot paraffin treatment that very day. I dipped my hands into hot, melted wax, withdrawing them to cool and harden. Moments later, the nurse removed the wax, and my hands indeed felt better and were less stiff.

"This works for rheumatoid arthritis," Dr. Brown chirped. "You probably have rheumatoid arthritis."

What? Didn't she know either? I wondered. Another round of medications. Another round of waiting to see whether they would work or not.

As I departed her office that morning, it dawned on me that I needed treatment more for my *knees* than for my *hands*, for goodness sakes. And my poor "beautiful, swollen knees" were still the same.

I gave this latest medical treatment a couple of months, with no success, and no resolution for the pain in my *knees*. She at last threw up her hands and said the words "Gold Treatment."

I couldn't afford to take off work every week for several hours for office visits, I told her. My job was hanging on the ragged edge, as my focus on my physical pain had caused me to make several minor errors on office paperwork, and The Sole Practitioner had given me warning.

I was once again Out of There.

A Few Words About Depression and Treatment,
or
The MHMR Marching Band

What I didn't know at the time was, I was in a depression, brought on by the disease itself. Anyone who deals with a chronic illness has a "built-in depression factor" and I was, indeed, "let go."

Once again, I'm out of work.

What am I going to do?

Why, find something else, of course.

In the meantime, I began a search to treat the depression that was descending on me like a shroud. My cognitive functions had deteriorated to the point that when I read something, I couldn't remember what I had just read.

Not a good thing in a working environment. Since I was unemployed, and virtually broke, I had to go to Mental Health and Mental Retardation Agency: MHMR. This would be the beginning of the Alphabet Jungle, consisting of acronyms such as TRC, WC, TWCC, and many other agency abbreviations.

I had a terrible time finding the place: First of all, the Summit Clinic is *not* on Summit Avenue. "Oh, it used to be, but they just kept the name when they moved," the clerk at the desk chirped.

MHMR was located, predictably, in the poorest, worst, "bad" part of town.

I parked my car in a junk-filled lot near vacant buildings with broken windows;

I emerged from the elevator to see a sign on the 2nd floor that says MHMR

But a cheerful clerk tells me I'm in the wrong place.

"Go up one more floor."

Grumbling to myself, and wondering what the hell I was doing here in the first place, I trudged up the flight of stairs.

I entered a gray waiting room where stale body odors assaulted me and sat gingerly in the on one of the gray-blue plastic chairs placed on soiled gray carpet.

It's miserably hot in here.

I read the signs all over the walls: "Do Not Park in the grocery store lot. Your car will be towed."

"Bring all meds with you to next appt."

Gray People shuffle in.

The Retarded. The Hostile.

Some tell silent jokes to themselves. Irritable mothers, hyper grown children.

The staff here deserves a medal

Finally, it's my turn to see the doctor.

He is weary-looking.

He asks questions.

"Every felt like killing someone?"

"Not yet."

He is not amused.
He scribbles on a pad.
I get a diagnosis.
"Adjustment disorder."
And a prescription for Pamelor.

As I am leaving, a nurse comes up to young man who is rocking back and forth, telling incomprehensible jokes to himself.
She hands his silent, drawn mother a bottle of pills.
"These will help his delusional states. Have him take two at lunch and two at dinner."
She says this right in the open. In front of everybody. Of course, there can be no secrets here.
Everybody here is crazy.
Except me.

Doctor #3

So I next went to work as a secretary in the management office of a large urban mall.
I lasted at that job about as long as I had lasted with Dr. Smith.
And I was still hurting.
I would try another job, and someone else, thank you.
That Someone would be Dr. Green. He more or less shrugged after extensive tests: "I don't find anything definitive." (A "diagnosis" I was destined to hear over and over again.)

Doctor #4

So I would be directed to University of Texas Southwest Medical Center. Surely at this prestigious teaching hospital, a diagnosis would be found.
Somewhere along here, it gets a little strange. (As if it weren't already strange enough!) I kept thinking about a woman I had known several years earlier. At odd moments, while I'm driving, not thinking about much of anything.
She had Lupus.
She had died of Lupus.

Why was I thinking about her? We were not close. We worked together at the Museum (as volunteers). In fact, I thought she was rather "crabby"---now I was beginning to see why.

Pain makes you crabby.

Why did I suddenly think of her? Could it be that I really did have Lupus, but nobody knows it but me? Does this mean I'm going to die?

"Not today," I muttered grimly, as I swung my car into the parking lot at UT Southwestern in Dallas.

"We tested you for SLE," the doctor told me. She was the finest rheumatologist around. Yet she said, "We found nothing conclusive."

How many times had I heard those or similar words "We can't find anything definitive."

. I returned to the law office where I had begun working after leaving the shopping mall job, diagnosis of "Connective Tissue Disorder" in hand.

Since I had spent more time out of the office than they felt was reasonable, I was summarily dismissed.

The journal entries begin. (Feel free, by the way, to skip over parts you aren't interested in, or feel like you've read it before. Sometimes I repeat myself: Lupus Lapse.

I decided to keep a journal reflecting my daily bouts with the disease of Lupus. If you think there are an enormous amount of entries, you should have seen those that I cut! Many seem repetitive, but that's what I was feeling at that time in this battle with Lupus.

I chose to personify this disease with the name of "Lupe" – and she takes on the persona of a gypsy, moving at whim throughout my body, setting up camp some days in my knees, other days in my wrists…and always, she builds campfires, stoking them, tending them carefully, unmindful of the pain these fires are causing me.

Lupe is actually a quite remarkable woman. She is vivacious, fiery, (pardon the pun), flashy, an independent, gutsy sort of girl. Lupe has steadfastly refused to tell me why she has chosen my body to explore, nor will she listen to my pleas to vacate the premises. She just hums softly to herself, stirs the ashes of her campfire, and sits back to gaze into the smoke.

This past week, Lupe was in her finest hours. She traveled quickly, all over my body, building campfires and then moving on to a new spot. The weather was cold, sleet hitting the windowpanes, and the wind howled to get in.

Lupe was not, by God, going to get cold. She moved rapidly and her fires kept her warm.

3/18/88

There is a struggle going on inside myself. I don't know what it's all about, but I know it hurts.

I have been no stranger to pain these last two years. I wake every morning with the same disease I went to bed with the night before.... no miracles occurred during my restless sleep.

The physical pain will be there, I'm told, forever, unless or until I have a remission. And I can cope with the physical pain, I believe. Better than the accompanying depression that seems to cry out at night and to greet me first thing each morning.

I hurt. I don't want to move and make it hurt any more. *Depression tells me to stay still. Don't get up and go to work. Don't do your meditations, your reading, take the phone calls from your friends. Depression tells me I'm always going to feel used-up, burned out, crippled.*

Diagnosis at Last!
October, 1988

Job-wise, I kept taking the same action, expecting different results.

Went to temporary work, more of the same. Was put on the health plan, which led me to the doctor who diagnosed my baffling illness. Dr. Dunn. He asked me if I were part Indian.

"Yes, I am. My grandmother was half Indian."

He nodded. "North American Indians (or Native Americans) are particularly susceptible to Lupus. We'll get some blood work done..."

I sighed. Would there be anything to see? Another time of waiting, wondering and hurting.

The blood work came back.

And the little monster had shown up.

"It's Lupus."

"Thank God," I breathed. "Now we know what it is. Now we can treat it."

He told me my reaction was typical. After all this time…an answer.

I was prescribed cytoxan and prednisone.

Where There s a Will There's a Burial plot.

I tell my family I have Lupus – what it can do to me. They are puzzled, they are afraid. They are angry. They are helpless.

Except for my kids…they buy a burial policy for me. Not exactly what I would want as a gift, but I am touched.

However, it was almost a case of "too little, too late."

By February of the next year, I was in the hospital.

UNDATED:

I hate this disease. I feel like I don't deserve the pain and inconvenience it causes. I don't like being different from other people. I feel like a child who can't run and play with the other kids. I feel financially burdened, barely able to keep going, everybody wanting a piece of me and not enough of me to go around.

I'm scared, God. I think about dying a lot. Well, not a lot, but at odd times. I don't want to die because of this disease, thank you. If I had my way – I'd be an old lady in good health, who just passes away in her sleep

But I won't get to choose my manner of death. I can, however, choose my manner of living. I choose to live each day the best way I can. I treasure my friends, my family, and wish there were more time for them. I miss my children and wish I could be with them more. I have to remember that they have their own lives and not to burden them unnecessarily with my disease.

I want this Lupus to just go away and leave me alone. I want the doctors and medical bills and the blood tests to just fade away into oblivion. I want to bargain with God – think if I'm a good girl, He'll make me "all better." I also know God expects me to take care of this stuff as best as I can.

4/23/89

My doctor advised me that in order to help the vasculitis in my ankles I should sleep in lace-up, high—topped tennis shoes. I went to Wal-Mart and in the boy's department found some red and white high—topped tennis shoes.

The first night I put them on to sleep in, I was in misery.

It was summer. They were hot. I ended up kicking them off during the night.

This would never do. A friend suggested that I make a game out of it. Air-condition those dudes.

I ruined my manicure scissors cutting "vents" into the sides of the sneakers; then I cut Hearts and Stars all over, and on one shoe with magic marker printed "Wonder Woman" and on the other shoe "Shazaam".

One night, while getting ready for bed, I happened to see myself in the full—length mirror: it reflects this outrageous creature without my wig, thin, wispy black hair sticking out in odd directions from a nearly—bald head; moon face devoid of contouring makeup; un-mascara-ed eyes wide with fear; pale arms and legs incongruously thin against a thickening body bloated from prednisone ---a body that was clad in a white cotton gown with lace on the waltz length hem; and, beneath the flounce, *red, high—top boy's tennis shoes*. I gazed at this pathetic creature and it gazed back, and suddenly, I began to laugh.

And so did the reflection. We laughed until we were breathless, this crazed—looking woman, and then we trundled off to bed, wrestling the red, high—topped tennis shoes into position against the makeshift footboard, and falling into a deep sleep.

And that's when I knew I was getting better.

Somehow, I knew this was a sign of mental, if not physical, health.

Undated

I found a Lupus support group.

They asked us last night what makes us fatigued. Heck, I don't know! I don't even know when I'm tired until I drop over. I have to learn the early signs and stop before I get there. I'll have to ask someone to tell me.

Now I know…I'm not lazy. I am *tired*. Lupus makes me tired to begin with.

Worry makes me tired. (Money, moving, etc.)

Dishonest people make me tired…those who "blab" about nothing at all make me tired.

Procrastination makes me tired. The actual doing of the chore makes me feel better, actually.

Pain is the biggest fatigue producer. If I can stay out of the pain – fighting the pain is so very hard. I have to remember to take some meds for the pain.

Damn this disease. I don't want to go through what I'm going through. It's too much.

I have to grieve over my lost health. Part of me is gone. I'll never be the same again. Damn.

Today I begin Cytoxan.

I went into a rebellion yesterday afternoon. I don't want to do this. I want things to be "normal." But the reality is, I have a disease. The reality is, I must control this disease. I am not passive. I am not a martyr. I am not a "victim" of anything. I am a survivor.

So I took my Cytoxan.

The Texas Employment Commission Chorus

What a screw-up.

I was told to wait until my name was called. By 11:15, I asked. I was told, "You missed your turn when the 10:00 group was called."

I told them "I was told to wait until *my name* was called."

I finally saw a claims examiner, got chewed out because they didn't give me the correct print-out last time – (each examiner has his favorite print-out, it seems.)

I am to return on the 15th with my forms all filled out, etc. etc. If I were going to get sick, it would have been then.

I left and went to Social Security. Quite a walk with my cane, but I had free parking at TEC. Social Security was confusing, to say the least.

The Social Security Symphony in C Minor, or "You're Not Sick Enough"

The nearest I could figure out was, I needed to be sick enough to have not worked for a year, was not expected to get any better or was near death, before I could qualify for a disability payment of $500 a month.

Puhleese!!!

There is something very wrong here.

The upshot is, wait and see about my unemployment. If they contest it, then I'll file for disability & SSI.

I have no pride left. I'll do what I have to do to survive.

I have $10 in cash till I get a paycheck of some kind on the 15th.

I'm definitely into fear.

Undated:

I thought I would do God's will if He would just show me. However, I was thinking, *"I'll do God's will if he'll show me and if it fits in with my plans."*

All I knew is *I've been setting limits on God.* Let Him do for me what I cannot do for myself.

He always does so much better when I stay out of His way.

5/23/89 11:30 p.m
Another damn disease!

I found out today I have *diabetes*, too. That explains all the bladder problems and vision problems. I'm taking medication for the diabetes, now, too. I can handle it.

On the way home, I said out loud, in my car, *"Okay, God, so now I have another damn disease! If you've got anything else for me, why don't you give it to me right now, instead of stringing it out?"*

Fear overwhelms me when I think of my financial situation. What am I going to do? I need to work; yet I can't. It's all I can do some days to just stand up. I'm going to fall, or have an accident, or something awful like that.

I am not able, tonight, to write any more.

5/27/89
Dying is the Easy Part

I have finally realized what *Chronic* means. It will not go away.

I knew that in my head. Today I just know it.

I need to remember to stress *capability*, not *disability*.

Barbara, Nancy and Liz have ganged up on me. They have each told me they thought there was a time there when I didn't want to live.

They were right.

Some days I feel that way.

But today I have a goal.

I feel very strongly about writing a novel. Maybe that's what I need to be doing. It's just that there are so many things that must be done first.

God, give me direction.

I talked to Carmen a long time. She said she thought for a while I had chosen death instead of life. I don't know when the turning point came, except I just got angry and decided to let that anger work for me.

5/31/89 5:50 a.m

Today, I start taking Micronase. 2 at 2x a day. I am in fear about that. At least until I talk to Dr. Morton. Will pick up the lab slip this a.m. and go to TEC for Federal job listings.

I am in such a grief process. I am losing my house. My income is almost nil. Really crappy day. But I got into expectations. And I can't expect anything.

6/4/89 Sunday

I am tired and frustrated.

Dad doesn't know how to treat me anymore. He either hovers or is distant. Mom is almost the same way. They just don't know what to do with me, now.

I need to tell them more often – I need to tell Mom "I can do this" or "I need help with this…" don't make them guess.

6/5/89 –5a.m

Sometimes I just have to cry.

I'm grieving my past life. For all the things I thought I needed – really, wanted – and it hurts to give things up. But things are just that. Ideas are painful to give up…the idea that I am someone other than who I am…I always thought I was such a proud person independent, sassy, even vengeful. Able to take care of myself.

Now I'm finding out I can't be that way anymore. I must depend on others. I must give up some things. I'll have a garage sale, move to an apartment. The house is just a house. I'll make a new home for myself. Heaven knows I've done that before.

But first I have to grieve.

I swing out of one mood into another. Pessimism to optimism. It's partly the meds.

Nobody has an easy life. It just looks that way to me. Now I'm having to find out who I really am.

6/6/89

I am just now realizing the dreadful power of this Lupus. It has wreaked havoc in my life and I'm angry. The things it could do to me further infuriates me… I could have more major organ involvement. I could go blind – have seizures – no telling!

I pray for health, for a job, for a place to live.

I pray for all those dear to me, and for my enemies.

I pray to live through this day.

6/9/89

I've been almost isolating. It's easy to do. But I know I'm better off among people, most of the time. Then I can rest.

Am going to the Women's Center this a.m. and check out the job leads. Maybe I can find a piddly little job. Dear God, guide me in the direction I need to go.

HATS

One straw hat
Started it all.
A fun thing to have,
To wear with a flair.
On hat led to another
And then there were three.
Might as well discover
What others there might be.
Wal- Mart has dozens
And the price was right, too.
I picked up "several"
Red, yellow, and blue
And black, and another straw hat
And did I have fun!
Almost like playing dress-up
I thought I'd never be done.
I wore my blue hat today…
I must say I looked chic.
It gave my spirits a lift
Compliments I didn't seek.
But I got them, anyway,
And it made me feel just great.
Thank you Lord,
For little things –
Like blue straw hats
And a sunny day
And the courage to face my infirmities
With grace and humor and strength.

6/20/89 a.m.

I am feeling overwhelmed again. And fearful. I'm afraid I won't get a job. I'm afraid I won't have any insurance. I'm afraid I won't survive.

I'm afraid of myself.

I'm afraid that if I don't get a job soon, before unemployment Insurance runs out, I will commit suicide.

36

Those thoughts have entered my mind. I don't want to, but there seems to be no way out…Just die and get all this mess over with.

Life has been so tedious at times. I know it's wrong thinking about wanting things to go smoothly all the time. But I don't see, dear God, why I have to go through this. Are you testing me? It seems I've struggled so long. I'm **so** tired of my life being **so** difficult.

6/27/89 Thurs.

I received in the mail an American Express money order for $100.00 Plus $10.00 in cash. Anonymous, of course.

My publisher at the newspaper called and said if I could deliver next week's column on Wednesday, she'd give me my check early.

The Realtor and his wife came by to appraise the house and sign a contract. He noticed my Al-Anon literature and asked me about my religion.

I sidestepped and said I was more spiritual than religious, and I said, "I know God sells houses."

He then told me of his experiences in seeing the sick healed. Said he had been praying for me and would work with me any way he could. And before they left, we stood and held hands and prayed.

Rather, they prayed.

I blubbered.

God certainly brings people into our lives just when we need them.

8/7/89
Spirituality vs. Religiosity

My Realtor and his wife invited me to a healing service the next Sunday ——— at a charismatic church.

Well, I'm Episcopalian, and was hesitant, but I figured, what did I have to lose?

These people spoke in tongues. They waved their arms and danced around.

God, I breathed, please don't let me get up there and faint and flap around like I've seen them do on TV.

And then the service was over and everyone was leaving.
All but us.

An elder of the church approached me and asked, "Do you want to be healed?"

I nodded and he led me to the front of the church, where no one was paying the least bit of attention to me.

Good.

He showed me passages in the bible that told of healing miracles and asked if I believed.

I nodded again.

He asked us to pray and then he took a vial of oil from his pocket and made the sign of the cross on my forehead.

Well, this Episcopalian lost it.

I bawled and squalled, and I don't cry pretty.

But I didn't fall down and flop around.

He then told me that I might not be healed right now. It may be next week. It may be next month or next year, and I might want to come back again, but, he assured me, "You will be healed."

We left and went to lunch and they took me home and about two weeks later I noticed I didn't have to use my cane.

9/11/89 Monday a.m

I'm tired of fighting life. I'm tired of taking medicine that doesn't seem to do a hell of a lot of good.

I'm tired of fighting government bureaucracy, of filling out forms, of "justifying my existence."

I'm tired of people giving me advice.

I'm tired of people asking me if I have a job yet.

I'm tired of people asking me how I feel.

I'm tired of feeling like a criminal because I'm ill.

I'm tired of this disease.

What more can I do? My therapist assures me that I'm doing everything humanly possible to help myself survive. Yet it seems useless. Nothing is happening. I'm running into brick walls. What are my options?

Give up and live on disability –if it comes through. That seems appealing at times. Just sit back and let 'somebody" take care of me.

It's too much, God.
I'm tired of it all.

11/29/89

Am I supposed to just "survive" and not have any goals? Nothing to strive for, no aim or purpose, other than just to get through the day? One day after another? Can't I dream? Can't I plan?

I am so angry that this disease has robbed me of my plans. Never to know how I'll feel – what my health may be like – Christmas preparations have me "spinning" – what if? Well, what if? Christmas will still be here whether I am ready or not.

I'm feeling sorrow—grief – for my former self – my health – I want to tune out.

12/18/89
Shingle Bells, Shingle Bells….

As if Lupus, diabetes and vasculitis weren't enough…. I get the shingles, an affliction that I would suffer sporadically for the next few years. Pain on top of pain.

11/17/92

I just read what I wrote way back in Sept.
You'd think that things (and I) would have changed.
NOT! I still feel:
Less than, shame, fearful, deprived, restless, irritable and discontent, lonely, definitely so, at this time, resentful, jealous of others' possession, talents, and praise.
I'm tired of these feelings,

I'm tired of being poor – or of feeling poor. Not managing well? I need – God, you know I need to be able to make my bills (on time) and still have enough left over for medical emergencies, car repairs and a movie out, every so often, without feeling fearful.

2/14/93

My health problems won't go away. You'd think I'd be reconciled to them by now…I'm not "cured" but "healed" in spirit, at least. Making peace with Lupus at least most of the time.

"Surrender?"

"Retreat" is probably more like what I'm doing.

2/26/93 Friday

A thought. Why not work in the hospital temp pool and get on their HMO? And get prescripts paid for – or almost -- $5.00 per? Find out how much they'll take out of my checks…will it be worth it. Or, I could go to the county hospital.

3/8/93 – Monday.

Blue Monday. No work scheduled for today. So I'm "on the street", instantly. In my mind. Negative thoughts flood me. I feel constricted. Tight. Holding my breath. It's not healthy to do that, I know. I find myself almost paralyzed by fear.

I sit beside the window and look at the tree. It's blooming. Bees gather around its blossoms. Birds are building nests. The tree is not concerned about anything. God planted it there and it's just doing what a tree is supposed to do – bloom in the spring, give shade in the summer, shed leaves in the fall, and endure the winter.

My "winter" is gone. It's spring. I'm alive. Perhaps not living an ideal life, but alive, nonetheless.

I've been in worse spots than this, and walked through it. I remember when I was in the hospital. Fired. Looking for a job while carrying a cane and wearing a wig and going home each day crying with pain from my swollen legs…rubbing ice on them. God carried me thorough that time…why do I disbelieve now?

I need to grieve. I need to rage. I need to cry for my soul. I have been wounded in many ways, over many years.

I feel my energy is not being focused, but scattered. What is important? What is necessary? What do I need right now? Rest? Probably. I have drawn on my reserves too often, like an overdrawn bank account. There is not much left to draw from. But

I ask: "Is it Lupus or is it life?" Is this normal to feel so down and discouraged?

I will get through this. And come out stronger.

11/12/94
Asthma?

Why am I still struggling with my health when I'm supposed to be in remission?

A trip to the ER early Thursday morning once again shows me that I'm vulnerable.

ASTHMA? Isn't it enough to have Lupus, diabetes, high blood pressure – what the hell am I doing now with ASTHMA?

I can't stop living in order to live. I have plans for my future. And these plans do not include illness. I have been called stubborn; that's not all bad. Another word is perseverance. I know what is important to me, and by God's grace I will do it. I am doing it. I've been through much worse than this.

I have much to be grateful for. My friends and family. Their concern and help.

My fear is that something so trivial might kill me. More than that, I might die before I've accomplished my tasks here on earth.

Surely God has a reason for my being here.

10/31/96
Trick or Treat!

Halloween –

Found out last Friday that ol' Lupe is back. In my pleura. "Lupus Pleuritis" is officially diagnosed. After all the howling I did at the clinic – the x ray showed it.

I was told by an intern, who dismissed my symptoms. I asked for my regular doctor.

No, I **demanded** to see my regular doctor. He assured me this is just a flare. But I feel so tired. Like I did before. The main thing is to keep from getting pneumonia. So I'm on antibiotics and high doses of prednisone.

At least I'm not hurting really bad. And the coughing has almost stopped.

But I'm still angry that it took so long to realize I'm having a flare. And I'm just plain mad that it's back!

Lupe must be pleased. She waited and softened me up, lulled me into a false sense of security–

I trudge on.

But damn, I'm still mad.

11/20/96

Still feeling kind of tired. So grateful that I've dodged the bullet, though.

I'm almost glad I'm not going back to school next semester. It will be cold, dark, dreary – the long drive and the studying – I don't need that at this time in my life.

Am I wrong in thinking I don't need any more stress than necessary at my age? After all, I have to be realistic.

What are my needs?

My needs are being met.

1/12/97

Not much change. Have a bad upper respiratory infection – again—got an antibiotic. Will take it for 2 weeks then have blood work done at Dr. Marsh's. She doesn't think it's Lupus.

I wonder.

Life sucks. And my attitude right now

It's snowing. I'm warm, semi-well. I still have lights and heat and food. And family and friends. This, too, shall pass.

But I want it to hurry up.

March- April....

I broke my arm in Discovery Training in Dallas. Fell out of a chair. Had to leave the conference. Broke my "write" arm. DAMN!

5/3/01 Friday p.m.

Changed meds again. Dr. K. said Effexor, 150 mg. Is what I need now. Tapering off the Paxil. Also got another sleep prescription.

Damn! The broken arm sent me into another downward spiral. Increased Paxil – didn't help. I just was back in the pit. No energy. No joy. Didn't want to go anywhere. Can't write.

My "raison d'etre" was taken from me. Suffered from the criticism at Writers Roundtable Conference in March. May 7, 2001

Need to write. Arm still hurts, though.

DAMN! My Counselor told me this would be a rough time…between meds. Between depression and recovery. "Between the devil and the deep blue sea."

10/19/2001
Much has happened.
Too much.
September 11th. Oh, God.
The Twin Tower/Pentagon attacks seemed unreal. I also haven't worked since then. Many others are out of work, for real. I asked the temporary agency for more work. So far, an offer of temp to perm, but I can't do that.

I take a trip to Alpine TX, with my mother's family, to explore the grounds where I was born.

Oh, and btw….I'm being published!

Here Endeth the Journal
Today, I'm okay.
Not "cured," but better
Gradually, year-by-year, I have been recovering. I've had six books published and moved again. I know Lupus will never be entirely defeated. At best, I can arrange a peaceful coexistence with this wild gypsy Lupe who runs about setting smoldering campfires in various parts of my body.

I expect that some day I will have another flare, but so far so good. If I can manage my stressors, gut enough rest, follow doctor's suggestions I'll continue to do well — and try to help others through the Lupus Foundation of America.

While I was a darn good secretary, this was not my "calling," and at my last place of employment, I vowed that I would not spend the rest of my life working to make somebody else rich, adhering to arbitrary rules and procedures , in short, I would find work that meant something to me, personally, that my soul had been seeking.

You can call that impractical, but to me, it's part of what had made me ill in the first place.

That inner voice that kept telling me I was in the wrong marriage, the wrong job; but fear had kept me from taking action.

After facing Lupus, I had no fear left.

To paraphrase Pogo, "I have seen the enemy and it is me."

Most of the time, Lupus is far from my mind.

And always, always, I pray that I never forget what this disease has taught me.

To be patient with others;
To be humble before God and my fellow man;
To be compassionate with those less fortunate;
To treasure every moment of every day;
To stay in The Now;
To know that in the end, it's just me and God.

Now, Some Stories and Messages from Other Lupies

When I became too ill and fatigued to attend a local Lupus support group, I turned to the Internet and found a yahoo group called "LUPIES."

Here was another way to get support and information. I began skimming through the message board, wondering if it would be worthwhile to commit myself to this anonymous group of women. I discovered a pleasant surprise:

These women, from all over the globe, (Australia, Canada, Philippines, and Texas (lol) are bright, articulate, compassionate and knowledgeable about this disease, even if much of it comes from their own experiences in dealing with SLE. I must add here that occasionally, a male of our species wanders into the group, and of course, he is welcomed. However, they are few and far between, and many times, it seems they have found the information they are looking for, and they no longer post. So, Lupus is mostly about women.

They shared their experiences, bad times, good days, vented about uncaring health care professionals, helpful and unhelpful relatives, and how they cope on a daily basis with this enigmatic illness, where there seems to be no set pattern of progression, methods of achieving remission and recovery, and how badly they miss the women they were before Lupus.

I laughed, I cried, I empathized. I then began posting about my own experiences; the good, the bad and the ugly. We found common ground in being disappointed with the vast majority of the medical community who seem surprisingly unaware of how Lupus can be diagnosed and treated. In other words, I say with tongue in cheek, we have a common "enemy" besides SLE.

After belonging to this group for about a year, I proposed to the owners of the list that I wanted to re-write my first book about Lupus, this time incorporating messages from our membership. Those who cared to participate were sent a Contributor's Release for signature, agreeing that I could publish their remarks. The owners, Sandra, Barb and Mary Mike, agreed, and I began revising my first book, and adding comments from Lupies.

As I read the heartfelt entries and tried to assign categories for ease of reading and understanding, I found that many of the entries contained remarks about several issues at once…. We are sick people, looking for help and understanding about many issues, and many times, they are all rolled together, like an enchilada on the menu of your favorite Mexican food restaurant. Or at the Chinese Buffet: One from Column A, One from Column B.

We really don't have an Al la Carte Menu. You take what is given.

So, here are some of the entries taken from our Lupies support group over a two or three year period. Looking at unsorted, impossible to categorize messages will be like a treasure hunt for the reader. You may stumble across something that you recognize as being exactly how you feel, or you learn some new information about this disease.

I have permission documents signed by the participants, so they know their words will be quoted as written, from the heart, with only an occasional edit by the author. The reader will notice that some posts are longer than others; and that a few people post regularly.

I'm not playing favorites by choosing the messages for this book. Some Lupies are more verbal than others. Some drop in only occasionally, but with great insight to a newcomer's questions. The only "rule" is: All of the participants have Lupus or are suspected as having Lupus, and are willing to write to others and expose their feelings, their pain, and their depression. They also offer hope, and "helpful tips" on coping, or small notes on alternative medicines.

Each person is welcome to the group for their experience, strength and hope. And, yes, for their complaints, rants, thoughts of suicide, and other issues. Sure enough, the moment someone posts that they want to "give up," several others add their voices of "me, too!" and relate how they got through that particular phase of grief.

Yes, grief. We have lost our former selves. We have lost our jobs. We have lost or alienated our families and friends. We deny, we bargain, we finally accept. That doesn't mean we like it.

I also noticed postings that said, more or less, "You play the hand you are dealt. It does no good to ask for different cards, a re-shuffle, so to speak. You were dealt a hand you didn't ask for. It doesn't matter whether you wanted it or not. It's yours. Now, make the best of it."

I hope you gain some insight into this disease, whether it is yours or you are reading to understand a loved one's struggle. God bless you if you are. We need support through this process that is ever changing, ever challenging, and ever-misunderstood.

Living with the Wolf:

Living with Lupus has been likened to "living with the wolf." Like the wolf, Lupus is hard to capture and tame. No matter how well you think you have Lupus under control with medications, sooner or later, "the wolf" eventually reaches out and takes a bite out of your life

Like wolves, each Lupus patient is different. Some have few symptoms, and have an outward appearance of being healthy. While others have so many symptoms of the disease, they feel like the proverbial "road killed wolf."

Being diagnosed with Lupus no longer deserves the "death notice" disease as it once did. Now the disease is better understood. It is more easily diagnosed with newer blood profiles thus enabling treatment to begin sooner lessening the damage done to internal organs.

Yeah, I got the same speech a couple of times about complement levels. I just stare at the doctors and blink when it comes up now... as if to say, "Okay, what do you want me to do about it?" It's not my fault the disease isn't cooperating with their standards.

The human body isn't a textbook or a computer app that you can tailor to a profile. Sick is sick. Lupus doesn't magically dissipate because some blood test doesn't look the way they want it to. Some of us also have high, rather than low, platelet counts. They don't want to talk about that, either.

Tala

A New Normal:

Gretchen:

I was told by somebody very wise that we have to establish a "new normal." What we did yesterday doesn't matter today. Today, it may be all we can do to get out of bed, and that's okay, for us. For that day. Yesterday, we cleaned the house. Today, it's all we can manage to load the dishwasher, and then go crash. That's a new normal.

You're going to grieve over your old self. What you used to do, what you used to feel like. Missing the sunshine, but realizing it is harmful to you. It's a process of adapting to what is, rather than what should be.

We're here to help you get over the speed bumps. Or, in our cases, the "slow bumps."

Marilyn

I Am Newly Diagnosed as Mild SLE...Is Anyone Willing to Share Similar Experience?

Hi, Kelly, and welcome.

Many of us started with mild symptoms, but others with severe and sudden onset of symptoms. Lupus is a disease that is unique to the individual patient. No two patients have the same onset, timing, intensity, variety, or appearance of symptoms. Many of us have symptoms in common with others, but no two cases are ever identical. This is what makes it so hard to diagnose and to treat. For instance, my test results have vacillated between positive and negative for over thirty years, now.

My current rheumy has no sense of humor and no depth of thinking, so I have to pretty much fend for myself. I have to insist on treatment, and since my meds work for me, it's very hard for him to try to change my medication routine.

Also, I have other indicators which make it kind of impossible to deny: blood disorders, sun related skin problems, fatigue to the max, low grade fevers, mild Sjogren's, heart/kidney involvement, etc. etc. etc.

So, in answer to your questions: We can't know what to expect from Lupus, but we CAN slow it down and make ourselves more comfortable.

Get started on Plaquenil as soon as possible as it can take up to six months to kick in fully.

Keep posting to this group for answers, support, to laugh or cry, or even whine (We offer cheese with that.)

Know that you are not alone in this. We have all been in your shoes, and we know all about how it feels. You can safely talk to us via this group, and get responses from anyone who is well enough to reply.

MM (Mary Mike)

Lab Tests

Dear All,

I must first tell everyone in this little chunk of cyber-land, thank you. I don't post much because I have dial-up Internet, it hurts to type, my brain is stupid, it is exhausting to stay focused...need I go on?

I wish that I could be sunshine and roses today. But alas, I am not. I have had a horrible day. It started when I had to start motivating my reluctant, achy body to move at 5:30 am only to drive 90 miles to undergo my third MRI this year.

After being stripped of my clothing and given the thinnest gown and sent into a freezing cold room, where the tech tried 3 times before finding a vein for the IV. I was then placed face down, on a board that had cut outs for me to place my breasts. Needless to say, the board was made of some material that felt like limestone, and I'm so small that my breasts didn't fit in the holes properly, so the tech had to "manipulate" them into position, which made me cry.

THEN, the tech placed my arms above my head and placed my face in a circular holder that raised my head up just enough to make my neck feel like it was in a vice and kept my breath from escaping, so all I could breathe was my own carbon dioxide. Get this picture... I've got all this going on and they place headphones with blaring music on my head and push me inside a tube making sounds like you have a helmet on your head and someone is hitting it with a hammer FOR OVER AN HOUR!!!!

The tech stopped twice and told me that I had to control my body motions and stop breathing so quickly or she was going to stop the procedure and I would have to come back another day. What part of *seizures* don't they understand? What part *of my whole body hurts, or I'm noise sensitive,* don't they understand?

Or how about this one? I just got over a fight with thyroid cancer, and I have:SLE Lupus and now I have lumps in my breast that are looking suspicious and I am scared to death, don't they understand? WHY DOESN'T ANYONE try to understand? I may look fine on the outside, but my insides stink.

I'm sorry for the rant. I know I'm crying to the choir, but I am tired, I'm hurting again, and I am scared. It seems I take one step forward just in time for the rug to be pulled out from under me. I just want to be a normal person. UGH.

Beth

I think I need a cane....

Ditto to Georgia's advice re: a cane. Without the rubberized bottom/tip your makeshift cane is going to slip around easily and you risk falling. It also isn't properly sized for you to use it correctly. I keep one in the car and one in the house "just in case" tho' I rarely use them. On bad days, when I was first diagnosed and before meds began to kick in, I was using my office chair on wheels as a wheelchair to go from room to room - if, like me, you have no carpeting and one floor that might be an option for you as well.

Ditto also to Freecycle advice. You'll see after a while there are greedy people saying, "I want" but also many truly in need. And many generous people who are glad to keep things out of landfills and see continued use. I've seen everything from drinks and food that people bought to try and didn't like right on up to clothing, computers and accessories to washers, dryers, pianos and TVs.

Sue M. in W PA

Eczema and Lupus of the skin

Christel,

I have some discoid symptoms, patches of skin that look like psoriasis, but which also can look like dry tiny blisters, bruising, large blisters that swell and burst. It's so much fun. NOT. Anyway, when they are all done, they leave behind no pigment whatsoever, and those white, white places are more susceptible to skin cancers.

I wear long sleeves, driving gloves when I am not able to use sunscreen, and wear large, shady hats. I have one that is considered a medical device, but it has no style, and is not the sort you can put a ribbon on, or anything. So, I stick with closely woven straws.

I found that most skin lotions do not agree with me, either. So, I make my own preparation of 2-3 parts Bag Balm mixed with 1 part Cortaid ointment. I mix it in the palm of my hand, and gently apply it to my rashes, lesions, et al. It helps heal, stops itches, and can be used repeatedly without ill effect.

Loving hugs,
MM

FFF:

--   Hi, everyone,

Bet you're wondering what the above initials stand for. How about "frustrated from fatigue." Just thought I'd get a rise out of everyone. Anyway, I have been pretty much attached to my recliner or bed for the past few weeks. I've gone out for my infusions and rheumy appointments but have stayed in pretty much since my trip to Ohio.

I started feeling a little better and collected some clothes for the Lupus Foundation pick-up tomorrow. Yesterday I had an appointment for my Yorkies to go to the groomer. I dropped them off, went to the pharmacy for $300 worth of prescriptions, picked up dog food and stopped at Bed Bath and Beyond to get a Brita water filter. Picked up the dogs and pulled into the garage just in time before the thunderstorms started.

I am so exhausted today I can't even describe it. This is the worst ever. I just want to sleep and drink water.

Thanks for letting me vent. Hugs to everyone,
Donna N.

I feel cheated..

Call your referring doctor and tell him just what you told us. Then ask for another referral, and, in the meantime, see if he would prescribe something for your pain. There's no reason anybody should tell you you're NOT in pain when you obviously are.

Your primary doctor suspects you have Lupus, but this "specialist" does not? GRRR! Lots of us Lupies never have joint pain, but our kidneys or lungs get attacked. Lots of us Lupies never have the discoid rash, either. There is no "one size fits all" for us.

Don't put up with this "doctor's" b.s. What I'd like to see is when a competent doctor finally does something for you; go back to this jerk and slap your medical file down on his desk (a copy, of course) and tell him sweetly, "I thought you might like to see this."

A thought, too. Is there a teaching hospital nearby? These new doctors are willing to go the extra mile to diagnose a patient (*House* notwithstanding!) so they can get brownie points from their supervising docs. I went to a local clinic of a teaching hospital and got excellent treatment.

Let us know. We're with you....

Marilyn

Kiki,

Thanks for the kudos, honey, but it's to keep my spirits up as much as anyone else's. LOL Helping others cope is how I cope. Comes with the territory of being the eldest in a large family, and not just eldest in my immediate family, but eldest girl of 56 first cousins. Yipes! Hahahaha.

I find it best to not obsess over what may be, but get ready for it and then forget about it. It just takes too high a toll on us Lupies to stress out over stuff. And, I believe, in fact, that stressing out is one of our worst symptoms. I was not a worrier before I got sick; I sort of went with life's natural ebb and flow.

However, once all this autoimmune stuff came to a head in my twenties, not isolated odd symptoms, but the whole magilla, I found that I was under more stress than ever, and most of it by my own hand, so to speak. I worried about every hiccup. Then, I started to notice how stress, emotional upset, or "nerves" were making matters worse for me.

That's when I started looking for ways to relieve stress, mellow out with visualization techniques, and to return to my former view of life as a natural sequence of events that we all experience in one form or another.

Nobody is exempt from life's strains, but they can make it easier on themselves by giving over to someone or something else each day. I write my worries and fears down on paper. When I feel I have expressed whatever it is that is bothering me, I make a ceremony of destroying the notes, and give it over. My motto is: Let the paper worry and twitch; I don't need this nervous itch.

Works for me almost 90% of the time. When it doesn't work, I know it's more important to me than I thought, and I rethink the situation. THEN, I let the paper have it.

I believe this is why I have survived this disease and complications for over 30 years. Of course, I AM stubborn as a mule, too. LOL

Loving hugs,
MM

Good News!

I have good news that I wanted to share. I have been in a horrible flare for almost three years and to tell you the truth, four months ago when I started having seizures along with all of the other Lupus complaints, I wanted to throw in the towel and just end my misery. I have been taking Lexapro, synthroid, Plaquenil, steroids, taking steroid shots, tramadol, xanax, nexium, and 800 mg Motrin for two years with limited progress. I've tried a host of other medications along the way but the side effects were just too hard to handle.

Three months ago I started taking Imuran and within 3 weeks I started being able to move around without making grunting noises, three weeks later I could actually blow dry my hair without crying, and yesterday I actually went to the grocery store by myself. I'm still a long way from being anywhere close to normal and I still have all the classic complaints, BUT...they are at a much less intensity.

For the first time in three years I am feeling encouraged. I am able to tolerate the Imuran without any of the major side effects as long as I take it with a full meal and I wash it down with a bottle of Ensure. I know Imuran is a horrible drug and the side effect is lymphoma, but I had no quality of life and at least now I actually feel like I'm in the world of the living. Has anyone else had significant improvements on Imuran?

Beth

Medical Alerts and Devices

While reading your post, I was reminded again of what would happen to us if we were by ourselves and had an ER visit while unconscious, or at home alone and fell, or any other dire consequence. ....

I wear a medic alert bracelet, available at any drugstore. I bought it mostly for medics/others who might find me unconscious from a low blood sugar dive (I'm insulin dependent diabetic.) Fortunately, the one time I was almost unconscious (while driving, shudder) I was able to tell the Highway Patrol man who pulled me over 50 miles from home (don't have a clue how I got there) from driving 25 mph on the Interstate. I blurted out -- lord knows how I managed to be that coherent -- "I'm diabetic and I don't know where I am." He called paramedics, rooted around in my car for any kind of sugar, found a peppermint and told me to put it in my mouth. He stayed until the paramedics gave me glucose (vile tasting tube of gook) and he agreed with them I should be taken to the nearest ER for a checkup.

Anyway, I wish now I had had the medic alert bracelet. I'm thinking of adding to the information "SLE" in case I'm ever in another situation like that.

And my son bought me a pendant from Radio Shack that he programmed into the telephone -- if I ever do the "help, I've fallen and I can't get up" thing, all I need to do is press the button on the pendant and the phone calls my son. If he doesn't answer (I can talk to him on the phone from over 50 feet away) then it dials the next name on the list, and so on, and the last one is 911.

Marilyn

Allergies, Disability and Antibiotics

Gerri,

You sound like me, honey. I spent today between my doc's offices at Kaiser having him fill out disability papers, for the twelfth time in twelve years...yeppers, every year like clockwork. Like there is going to be this miraculous cure. Idiots! Anyhow, I told him to tell the people that I am from another planet: The planet Lupus, which hovers somewhere in mid-galaxy struggling to avoid the sun.

I sure hope your rheumy finds some answers for you, and tells those idiots who want to test you on drugs to take a long hike off a short pier. I, too, am allergic to a raft of antibiotics, have had reactions ranging from rashes to anaphalaxis, to fainting, red lines on my arm from an IV site moving toward my heart, etc. Life in the Lupus Lane is a real roller coaster ride. They tried giving me iron by infusion two days ago, and I had a bad reaction to it, so therefore, transfusions are coming up. Ick.

Sending you soft, warm hugs,

MM

I am having a terrible time! Any suggestions?

To those experiencing weird reactions to meds, and other stuff:

Allergies, smallergies! I think part of having autoimmune disorders is that we react weirdly to all things.

Meds that are meant to relieve pain often promote it, pills for relaxing and sleeping often keep us awake, antibiotics can backfire on us, and anti-inflammatories can eat holes in our digestive systems. Sheesh, can we get any more complicated as a patient group? Oh, yeah, and we each present as uniquely as fingerprints in an FBI file. Double Sheesh!

Do others in this group have these experiences? Well, I ask you my loves, do we? YOU BET! Did I spend five days in ICU last October because of a deadly reaction to the H1N1 shot? Yeppers. We Lupies are a real bundle, and we get more complicated with every little thing science learns about the disease. All I know is that I am sick and tired, and sick and tired of being sick and tired, and sick and tired of being sick and tired of being sick and tired...ad infinitum ad nauseum.

Love you all,
MM

Re: Doctor Appointments

Not to overstate the obvious, but I see a lot of people post the same kind of problem, and.... you've got to put your foot down. While the Dr. is actually in the room with you, stop them if they aren't making sense and ask for them to use layman's terms along with technical so that you can both learn and understand what they are saying to you.

Explain to them that you wish to be an educated patient because you are aware that you are the one in charge of your own health care, not the Dr. You live in your body 24/7 and you're in charge at every given moment of what goes into it and how it is treated. They aren't at home with you - it is therefore critical that you understand what is happening and what your body needs. A lack of knowledge in an area like this can diminish your quality of life severely, and even end it. I'm sorry if that's blunt, but it's the truth. You must have information.

If they're acting like they are too busy, remind them that you're paying the bill. If you had to wait for them to show up (and I'm pretty sure in most cases, we all do), remind them that YOUR time is valuable, too, and that for someone who is chronically ill, the more time you have to spend on a task like an appointment, the more it costs you... in energy, strength, and well-being. If you've waited, then you deserve the Dr's full attention and assistance. It's their responsibility to do their ENTIRE job. If you have to remind them of that, then do it. For the record, no... they don't like it. You know what though? WHAAAA! I don't really care if they like it or not. I tell every Dr I see when they're new that if I call, it's serious. I don't call about sniffles and bruises. I therefore expect them to take me seriously. The rheumatologist I see did just that (which is refreshing) and spoke to me like an educated adult, spending more time with me than he does with the rest of his patients and going over charts with explanations and discussion.

Five minutes *is not* an appointment. I would say that to the Dr in those words. Ask him when you should make your next appointment for that he will have the proper time for your needs. In those words. Two and a half hours of waiting is insulting, demeaning, unreasonable, and in my opinion, cause for reporting to various sources available re poor performance. I would never wait that long. I would be at someone's desk saying either see me now or tell me when to come back that the Dr can see me because I'm DONE. That stupid diploma doesn't give any Dr the right to treat you that way. Maybe you should go see him again and immediately ask the nurse for a blanket and pillow so you can take a two-hour nap till the Dr is ready.

My best advice would be to send a detailed letter explaining all of his errors in the situation, and find another Dr if you have the leeway to do so. Honestly. Your description horrifies me.

If they don't contact you when they are supposed to, then you have to let them know they've done wrong. If there is a medication you're not comfortable with then you deserve to be heard and offered options, or at least have an explanation about why there aren't any. There are almost always options and natural alternatives though... so do your own research on that as a backup - they don't always know, care, or divulge. Me, I research and inform the Dr myself.

Tala

Doctors

Welcome, Diane,

I'm sure we are all happy you found this site. It holds a wealth of information and understanding. I think most of us know how frustrating the process was until we finally found the cause of all of our symptoms and got a diagnosis.

Remember my Lupus prayer:

God grant me the serenity to accept the things I cannot change, the courage to change the things I can....AND THE WISDOM TO HIDE THE BODIES OF THE DOCTORS WHO SAID IT WAS ALL IN MY HEAD!!

Loopie hugs,

Donna N.*(Who asked me not to credit her with that prayer; she saw it on a T-shirt.*

Thyroid and Lupus:"

Dear Christine,

As the others have written and I am sure you have read, your story fits right in with many of our stories. My journey started much like yours. I became super sun sensitive, which started with a mottled, red skin rash and led up to fainting episodes when exposed to direct sunlight and heat.

I was first diagnosed with Hashimoto's thyroiditis and put on synthroid and just like you I had an energy level increase and my hair quit falling out. I thought my problems were resolved but two years later, I had thyroid tumors grow so fast that my students freaked out over how much bigger they had grown after a four day holiday.

I had my thyroid removed and all heck broke loose. I could not work nor could I do anything that required me to move around by myself. I struggled daily just to take care of my daily needs and every one and every thing in my life fell apart.

It took two more years before I was diagnosed with Lupus and 2 more years and here I am still trying to figure out what the heck is going on with my body. I too, can't sleep and have crazy dreams. My husband wakes me up frequently to tell me to be still or I wake up while he is wiping my eyes and holding me because I am crying.

When I asked my rheumy if I should be worried about my night time issues he sent me to neurologist who ran every test she had and still couldn't figure me out. The whole process of symptoms, diagnosis, and treatment is a huge boondoggle. Few answers, few solutions.

Sadly, I find comfort among those in this group who so sweetly listen to my trials and tribulations. I say sadly, because it breaks my heart that anyone else is going through this horrible journey. I wish that I had a magic wand that I could wave over you, me, and everyone else that crashes into the lupie world.
We are all trying to keep our heads above water. You are not alone.
Beth

How to get Family to "get it?"

If you've never been chronically ill, you don't know what it's like to wake up aching and debating about whether you have the energy yet to leave your warm blankets and stumble to the bathroom even though you really gotta go. If you've never had chronic pain, you don't know what it's like to have to - really HAVE TO - take your shoes off, get off your feet, and not get up again for several hours because you went to the grocery store for a few things. I know that someone with a healthy roll of luck in life can't grasp these things from the internal view of it... but it is possible to have compassion and concern without walking through it yourself.

I don't know what it is that makes some people so callous and self-absorbed. . and I'm really sorry that you and anyone else here have to deal with it. I know I do. That's what "awareness" is about, of course... so we just have to keep trying to get the information out there to people that will hear it. For whatever reason, family is the least of the listeners.
    Tala

Depression and Lupus:

Thank you for responding and telling some of the things you miss about YOU. I was in the beauty industry too, was a Sebastian Salon Rep, was a 'high end' cosmetic buyer, managed couture boutiques, modeled and designed...it was hard after being so creative and in such a FUN environment to be sent home to stagnate...I thought I'd die and was in such deep depression for a long time, wishing to die.

Like you, I have a wonderful husband...at first, w/out a DX, he wasn't understanding and we had some very rough times. I didn't know how to ask for help and hid a lot of my symptoms from him and my son because I was so scared and humiliated. . They thought I was having Menopause and thought I was being Bitchy, Lazy, Bipolar and Crazy and thought I could just 'stop it' if I cared to. My son was in Jr High when my symptoms got really bad and he was always so mad and angry with me.

I had become so depressed and suicidal, I didn't even try to explain the suffering, all the Drs couldn't 'find' anything wrong with me so they had my husband and son confused and wondering if maybe I was...crazy!...but I knew I wasn't and only GOD carried us thru about ten long suffering years of this, spending money we didn't have (we have no retirement because of this and have no college savings for my now 22yr old son)

Both of them are so wonderful now. My son came by the other day and just broke down in sobs when he went to hug me 'Goodbye', saying he had been a terrible son in those years and felt such remorse.

This terrible disease takes such a huge toll on ALL of us AND our families and friends, it's heartbreaking.

GOD be blessing you and your husband and I pray, Cyd, that soon we will be defeating this horror and that no one and their families have to go thru the suffering and the 'loss of themselves' as we did. Be blessed and be well...

Amen! Texas Carol

Here Are the 5 STAGES OF GRIEF

1. Denial and Isolation

The first reaction to learning of terminal illness or death of a cherished loved one is to deny the reality of the situation. It is a normal reaction to rationalize overwhelming emotions. It is a defense mechanism that buffers the immediate shock. We block out the words and hide from the facts. This is a temporary response that carries us through the first wave of pain.

2. Anger

As the masking effects of denial and isolation begin to wear, reality and its pain re-emerge. We are not ready. The intense emotion is deflected from our vulnerable core, redirected and expressed instead as anger. The anger may be aimed at inanimate objects, complete strangers, friends or family. Anger may be directed at our dying or deceased loved one. Rationally, we know the person is not to be blamed. Emotionally, however, we may resent the person for causing us pain or for leaving us. We feel guilty for being angry, and this makes us more angry.

The doctor who diagnosed the illness and was unable to cure the disease might become a convenient target. Health professionals deal with death and dying every day. That does not make them immune to the suffering of their patients or to those who grieve for them.

Do not hesitate to ask your doctor to give you extra time or to explain just once more the details of your loved one's illness. Arrange a special appointment or ask that he telephone you at the end of his day. Ask for clear answers to your questions regarding medical diagnosis and treatment. Understand the options available to you. Take your time.

3. Bargaining

The normal reaction to feelings of helplessness and vulnerability is often a need to regain control–

- If only we had sought medical attention sooner…

- If only we got a second opinion from another doctor…

- If only we had tried to be a better person toward them…

Secretly, we may make a deal with God or our higher power in an attempt to postpone the inevitable. This is a weaker line of defense to protect us from the painful reality.

4. Depression
Two types of depression are associated with mourning. The first one is a reaction to practical implications relating to the loss. Sadness and regret predominate this type of depression. We worry about the costs and burial. We worry that, in our grief, we have spent less time with others that depend on us. This phase may be eased by simple clarification and reassurance. We may need a bit of helpful cooperation and a few kind words. The second type of depression is more subtle and, in a sense, perhaps more private. It is our quiet preparation to separate and to bid our loved one farewell. Sometimes all we really need is a hug.

5. Acceptance
Reaching this stage of mourning is a gift not afforded to everyone. Death may be sudden and unexpected or we may never see beyond our anger or denial. It is not necessarily a mark of bravery to resist the inevitable and to deny ourselves the opportunity to make our peace. This phase is marked by withdrawal and calm. This is not a period of happiness and must be distinguished from depression.

Beth's Chronic Illness Stages of Thinking Over the Years

I read through the posts about the grieving process and I was thinking that the five steps didn't work for me. I started thinking back about my attitudes that I have had over the past 4 years and it is so complicated that I had a 12-step process. Here it is...

I somehow cut this from my previous post where I was talking about the five steps of grieving not fitting my situation. Here are my thought processes over the past four years of battling my illness. Take from it what you will.

Beth's Chronic Illness Stages of Thinking Over the Years

What is wrong with me?
I am not crazy.
Can I push past this?
What the h*ll is going on?
Why is this happening to me?
How many doctors do I need?
How can I swallow another pill or take another side effect?
What happened to my life?
Where did everyone go?
What is my new normal?
Will I be able to overcome my obstacles or
Is it time to surrender?

Well, there it is...my life in short form. I am sure I will add to my list, I ended it where I am right now.
Beth in Texas

Re: CNS Involvement:

Sometimes it is extremely difficult to explain to a treating physician why you are having a problem, what the problem really is, its severity, and why it is that you're so gravely concerned. They only see you for anywhere from 5 to 20 minutes, depending. That's on a day that you've planned a visit, rested, showered, eaten, and gone prepared to interact with other human beings for a purpose. We all know that it's possible to ramp yourself up for something like that unless you're in a severe episode/flare.

All the Dr. sees is a patient with a few complaints. They're accustomed to the basic case of 'take this pill and let me know if you're not better in a few months." They don't hear you saying it's been like this for X number of years already.

The biggest thing they DON'T see or hear is how **big of a change** it is and how it is affecting your life, your routines, your needs. If someone could never multitask, they aren't missing anything at 42 if they still can't do it. I, however,was an administrative assistant for the largest property management company in the state - a Receivership, in fact. I was a receptionist for multiline switchboards. I was a data entry clerk with 65wpm typing skills. I used to be able to get online and hold several conversations at once in chat, between a chat room and private messages, and keep them all straight WHILE posting on message boards. I would open windows and handle it all without batting an eye.

I can't. Not now. So if my norm was that kind of mental processing, then what I have now is severe damage for MY NORMAL. My PCP gave me that "mini mental" test recently and told me that I'm not demented. Well duh f***ing duh. If I were, would I be asking for help? Her test can't check on my personal baseline and it certainly isn't an in-depth examination. Just because I can remember 3 words in a setting where I have nothing else but the Dr to focus on, or can copy a couple of hexagons on a piece of paper with an example right next to where I'm drawing does NOT mean that I'm okay.

It was insulting.

What I'm telling you by sharing this much is that you're not alone. I think that most of the members here will tell you that your symptoms and difficulties are fairly typical, and are not always an indicator of anything deeper than "just the Lupus." The mental fog is overwhelming until you find personal ways to manage it. Then instead of being in tears at the store, because you can't find your car, you find moments at home to break down and have a moment... lol.

But at the parking lot, you can stand calmly long enough to be able to spot it. Let me make a suggestion to you about the car thing, though... buy one of those little bitty notepads (Wal-Mart has them, so does Big Lots for really cheap) and keep it in your purse with a pen. Write down when you park where you are. Most large stores like Wal-Mart even have aisle markers of numbers or letters. Scratch it out in the notepad once you are back in your car. If you might forget to scratch out or remove a page, write the date on it too. I've been through this more than I care to tell you... it's a lot.

Re not being able to find the right word, or get it verbalized.. . that too is pretty common in our situation. If for no other reason than chronic illness itself wears on a person, it's not all that strange for it to happen. It is, however, important that your care providers are made aware of it, how bad it is, and how distressing you find it. Don't let them dismiss it, certainly. I'm not.

The fact is, symptoms are there to tell us that something is wrong... and it could be something very wrong. You can't be sure. If it's a symptom that just won't go away or improve, then it deserves closer attention still.

In the mean time... your appointment and mine... all we can do is stop and take a deep, cleansing breath once in a while, okay? I know from personal experience that when you get into one of those moments of blank, and you can't recall what you need, the panic that sets in only makes it worse. Allow yourself the right to stand still and regroup if you need to. You're not required to perform anything in life up to *someone else's standards* of function. If you need to go slower, go slower.

Tala

CNS Involvement

Well, hell, Tala, if this is an example of 'impaired ability,' the REST of us are doomed!

I miss me too, no matter how well I've learned to adjust. I cry for the woman I was, cry for the safety and security I had in being me, cry for the beauty stolen and the strength taken and my mind, Gone. All vain things, of course, but even so, part of our feminine mystique and things I very much enjoyed. as a woman and going out into the world, just being ME!

Texas Carol

Normal Lupus Stuff

Welcome, welcome, Chris.

Until joining this group I had no idea that the things I experienced were 'normal' lupie stuff. Suddenly things just made sense. Even a lifetime of migraines seemed to be the norm. Lupie Fog was expected and I no longer worried I was getting Alzheimer's. Now instead of fear I just smile and shrug. All the NORMAL things took the back seat and I was and am able to look the enemy in the face and deal with the problem of the day. Some days not as well as others.

I love to laugh and this is a good group who laugh along with each other....cry, pray, worry and cheer one another on. We are like a hormonal pool of love.....lol I post some fluff but give fair warning in the subject line so just delete if you are not up to my nonsense. It will be great to get to know you.

Be well,
Val

Comment from doctors and a funny story

Everything I tell him that is wrong he just says "Well that's your Lupus." GRRRRRRRR what does that mean? That I have to live the rest of my life like this???

Gretchen

UUUUUUUGGGGGGHHHHH HHH!!!!! I hate it when a doctor says that! I agree...what does that mean? I have to put up with...or is he saying...get over it? I go from pleasant patient to mad lupie in 0.0 seconds when that comment is made to me. In fact, my husband and I now use the "its your Lupus" comment to lighten stressful events. For example, it took several swipes to get my credit card to work at a gas pump, and when my husband finally got it to work, finished filling up, and got into the car, I asked him what took so long and he said, "The card wouldn't swipe, it must be your Lupus." I laughed my butt off.

Beth

Re: Becoming Your Own Advocate

Dear Judy,

I have been exactly where you are in your Lupus journey. I was an active high school teacher and coach before all heck broke loose and I was diagnosed with Lupus. It started when I got every cough, cold, and illness in which I was exposed. Then I started having "female" issues and the dr decided to do a hysterectomy. I never recovered my previous energy level and felt lousy most of the time.

I then was diagnosed with thyroid nodules and had surgery to remove the nodules and the thyroid. I continued my downward spiral and with a positive ANA in hand was sent packing to a rheumatologist who ran more tests and was then diagnosed with SLE Lupus. This all happened within a four-year time span and somewhere in there, I gave up coaching to conserve my energy for teaching.

In October of 2008 my fatigue, pain, and continual battle with the Lupus playing with my heart, liver, and kidneys gave way to me taking medical leave. Although I don't miss the grading, paperwork, or Texas testing pressure, I desperately miss the kids and my love of teaching literature.

My journey has been marred by a host of doctors who did not treat my Lupus aggressively and my lack of knowledge of Lupus, and if I had it all to do over again, I would be a better advocate for my health. I am in fairly poor condition right now due to a battle with pericarditis and my cardiologist is convinced that I would not be in this sad state if I had pushed for more aggressive treatment.

It is sad to think that a chronically ill person must be in charge of pushing medical professionals, but, this is usually the case in treating Lupus. Since hindsight is 20/20, my goal is now to tell others my story in hopes that they will push for answers and treatment for their Lupus struggles. I hope that you find the right treatment quickly and that you can return to teaching.

Cyber hugs,
Beth

Will I ever have a pain free day?

Judi.

When we were little we would run to our moms and she would kiss our boo boos and that is all it took to make it feel better. As we got older the kiss didn't quite cut it and the big guns were needed....a bandage. But now we are all grown up and we realize, as you wrote so beautifully, that it isn't just about us, but about many who hurt and have had to work with a new normal that none of us want.

Many outside this disease do not get it and the advice they give is lame and at times, infuriates, but then, like you did, we post to our new normal family of supporters who really know, not only what we are verbalizing but also experience the pain and loss and everything else that goes along with this enemy. Lupus is an enemy but along with all of the others, we are learning tools to be able to tame and control and even embrace the wolf so that we can learn and grow and be even better than before. It is in tribulation that we will become stronger.

Will there be pain free days? Yes. Every day could be the one that the cure will be found or a medication that will have no negative side effects. Until that day we are a united voice who are here for each other with encouragement, prayers, hope, and friendship.

We are really quite fortunate, in that we are not alone; we have understanding and respect for where we are in our individual journey, shared with many who run alongside.

Be well
Val

A Name for our Illness:

I don't even like calling what we have a disease. *Illness* sounds nicer and I'm calling her Bertha.
Goodnite,
Georgia

Lupus Fog:

I cried and laughed through the Lupus fog postings. I know it shouldn't be funny...but sometimes you have to laugh to keep from crying. Recently, my daughter-in- law told me that she needed to talk to me privately. I thought...oh no. I started flipping through my memories of recent conversations with her trying to think of something my mother-in-law voice might have said, but I couldn't come up with anything.

I was so anxious about the whole situation by the time she got to the house I was sweating...I hate confrontations and usually avoid them at all cost. Besides, she is the only person in my life (besides my husband) who comes to my rescue when I have days that I can't get out of bed, and the thought of losing her friendship and help was too much for my already panicked brain to comprehend.

She finally arrived at the house and we talked over a diet cola. She had a tough time starting the conversation and finally just blurted out how concerned she was about some things I've said lately. She told me that I say the strangest things, I often start a sentence and stop because I can't remember what I was saying and that I never call people by the correct name, or remember events correctly, and that I often slur my words.

But the part that threw her over the edge is *when I called a butterfly a flying mushroom.* I laughed so hard I thought I was going to pee my pants. I remember the conversation, but I didn't remember saying *flying mushrooms.* She is 26 and I am 48 and I've known her for 13 years, but for the past six years she and my son have lived out of state and have spent a limited amount of time around me.

She remembers me as the mom, teacher, coach, and community leader that had it all together and took my academic teams to state every year. They recently returned to our hometown and live two blocks from my house and now spend almost every day around me. In the past two years my Lupus has been out of control and has settled into my brain. I haven't worked in a year because of my processing problems, but I don't talk about it much. It is hard enough to explain the pain I am in and my Lupus problems that no one can see and I sure don't want to burden others with my brain farts.

Anyway, she was mortified that I laughed and she was truly upset. We talked for a long time and I explained that this is who I am now and we need to keep track of the funny things I say just like we keep track of what my five year old grandson says. I tried to refocus her on the fact that she can't be sad, because it makes me sad and then my brain just shuts down. I am always better on the days that I laughed about my misstatements. I learned a big lesson from her and that is...sometimes you need to give people permission to laugh. Lupus brain fog is REALLY not funny, but I think it is my body's way of making it through just another part of this beast of a disease.

Beth

Lupus Fog

You said exactly what is in my head. I find I have a hard time putting things into words. It's like I've lost all my communication skills at times. It's so frustrating to have so much to say, but can't word it right to make someone understand. But you said this perfectly. I also find some one will tell me something & I'll forget it in a couple of days. So when I bring it up again, they look at me like I have a 3rd eye. When really I don't remember the conversation from the first time.

I too have gone through lots of pads of paper for reminder notes, & lost them too. I find the best thing is my cell phone. I put notes to myself in my drafts or on my calendar. This Samsung phone I just got has a place for notes & task. It has really helped me out.

For you being able to put into words what I couldn't makes you one of the greatest people to touch my life.

Hugs,
Naomi

Heidi's Story

I was diagnosed at 47 although thinking back I had symptoms before that. I am now 62 so I'm a veteran. I have a husband of almost 23 years, 2 grown daughters, 2 grown stepchildren and 7 grandkids. Two years ago we sold the big house in a northern NJ commuter town and moved to a slower moving town on the Jersey shore.

My official diagnosis is Undifferentiated Connective Tissue Disease (UCTD) with symptoms of subacute cutaneous Lupus, sclerderma and Sjogren's syndrome. I also have Reynauds and TMJ. My most recent setback was a diagnosis of lymphoma. Two months ago I had surgery to repair the tendons in my wrist that were scarred from the inflammation that limited the use of the fingers on my left hand. I'm a long-term prednisone and Plaquenil user. I take Cymbalta, Lipitor and Vit D supplements as well as calcium shots. Add in some Protonix for my stomach and Ambien to sleep. I've tried several immunosuppressants (most recently Methotrexate) with varying results. I'd say my health is relatively good.

So onward until my hand starts to hurt too badly or my computer battery runs out. I have 4 doctor appointments this week; thus my first topic.

Lupus is a Team Sport -- I attribute my relatively good health to the dedicated, knowledgeable, caring team of doctors I have assembled over the years. The other members of my Lupus team include my family and friends, both real and virtual.

So how did I get this team and who are the members? My first Lupus doctor was a dermatologist. I went to Florida with my husband for a conference in February 1994 and I enjoyed the pool while he was in meetings. I came home with an obvious rash on my upper arms. I went to a local dermatologist. She took one look at the rash and asked, "Do your joints hurt?" I said "yes" and she said she was pretty sure it was Lupus. She did a biopsy and phoned me with the results.....she was right about the Lupus. She would become my chief diagnostician, later diagnosing two cases of shingles and lymphoma. She referred me to a rheumatologist. He was the next member of the team.

I didn't know anything about Lupus so I did research. My sister is a diabetic so I initially thought Lupus wasn't as bad as diabetes and that I was lucky. I also did research on the rheumatologist. I also checked his hospital affiliation and his educational qualifications.

Following confirming tests we spent years developing cocktails of medicines. A known researcher in the field, the doctor relied on his expertise and consulted with other doctors to refine my medicines. Relying on prednisone and Plaquenil, immunosuppresents were added and subtracted and mixed in different combinations to improve my health.

All was well until 2001 when I had a fever of 105 degrees. At this point I did not have a Primary Care Provider (PCP) as I had fired mine after he missed the Lupus and a case of shingles. Since I was rarely sick, I relied on my rheumatologist to manage my care. I went to the ER and was diagnosed with pneumonia, placed on antibiotics and admitted to the hospital. The following day I had respiratory failure and I awoke in CCC 36 hours later. This incident added a pulmonologist, a cardiologist and an infectious disease specialist to my growing team. All were asked to see me by my rheumatologist who by this time had gained my trust and confidence. During this hospitalization I also acquired a PCP and his internist wife who are still part of my team.

A case of shingles in 2007 that infected my eye (leading to blindness in my right eye) added two opthomologists to the team....one specializing in retinas and one with a specialty in corneas. If recovering from shingles and the resultant 2 surgeries weren't enough, in 2007 I had a large lesion on the back of my leg that sent me back to the dermatologist. A biopsy identified the lesion as lymphoma. A referral from both the dermotologist and rheumatologist added an oncologist/hemotologist to my growing list of team members. Following a PET scan to ascertain the extent of the cancer, I was diagnosed with Non-Hodgkins lymphoma of the skin and left lung.

Two short-term team members include an oral surgeon (to remove my wisdom teeth) and an orthopedic surgeon who recently repaired the tendons in my left wrist.

So what have I learned? First, someone needs to coordinate the team. In this case it is my rheumatologist. What are the characteristics I look for? Respected by his peers, current with the research, plays well with others, listens to my concerns and issues, thinks outside the box, communicates in a timely manner, doesn't hesitate to refer me to others who know more than he does, and isn't intimidated by a second opinion.

Second, if a doctor doesn't meet my needs, I fire them. Third, good team members must communicate with me, each other and my rheumatologist. Fourth, I need to learn as much as I can about each illness, condition (or whatever I call it) so I can actively participate in my care and doctors on my team can't be intimated by a high maintenance patient.

Heidi

Brain Fog

Oh my goodness, Mary, how did you get into my head? Everything, and I do mean EVERYTHING you said about the fog is exactly how I feel every single day! I have a plaque in my kitchen that says, "Of all the things I've lost, I miss my mind the most". Wish there was something we could take to lift the fog but I guess it's not meant to be. I know this won't make you feel any better, but just know that you definitely are not alone in how you feel.

Oh btw, you didn't sign your post but I thought that maybe you couldn't remember your name lol so I searched for it so now we both know....of course I'll forget it within the next few minutes....oh well, It's like meeting new people every day haha gotta laugh; beats crying. I always try to find the humor in all the stupid things I do and it has been quite a source of entertainment.

Georgia

Brain Fog:

Thanks Georgia!

I am really wishing I didn't have to finish out the month right now but we need the money.

Writing about things always helps me too and it is great to have people here who understand what I am dealing with! ;-)

I get really teary during a flare too especially since I am prone to more mistakes and that really upsets me.

My daughter asked how to spell *Aunty* yesterday because she was writing on my niece's birthday card and I got to "t" and couldn't think what went next and said E! I got so frustrated and thankfully DH took over on that one! He saw me get upset over it and came and gave me a hug and said he loves me even more when I am like that because it's cute. LOL Glad he thinks so. To me it is just frustrating

I am petrified of losing my intelligence. I have been the sort of person that most things come easily to, particularly if they interest me and the thought of having difficulties with my mental abilities the rest of my life scares me a lot. Even more so than the pain, etc.

I console myself a lot with the fact that at least now that I have been fired from my job, I can do what I love most and that is designing, but what happens if I can't do that anymore. That thought really scares me, too.

I am hoping that the fact that my hours will be much more flexible and I can work pretty much as much or as little as I wish will mean that my flares will decrease and I will find things much easier. Plus the fact that designing isn't stressful to me, because I find it relaxing and I can just absorb myself in it almost like a good book.

Just rambling some more. to anyone who feels like listening.. Your input is of course welcome.

Robyn

Being Aware of Your Symptoms:

I was diagnosed with Lupus about one and half months ago and figure I probably had it for about 5-7 years.

I fear now that I am attributing everything to Lupus. I used to ignore my aches and pains and work through them most of the days. Now I feel like I feel things MORE than I did before..... but I also notice things that I believe I used to ignore, like brain fog, puffy face, dizziness, tightness in my chest, etc. In some ways I'm feeling a bit like a hypochondriac and of course no one I know really understands. I'm not a complainer, so I barely say anything to my husband although he's been really sweet and tries to remember to ask me how I'm feeling that day.

So does Lupus gain momentum? I look back at the last five to seven years and see all the signs. Some days I still feel like a "normal" functioning person and other days I wonder if I'm going downhill fast.

So now I think that just because my problems have a name, I'm thinking about it all the time. It's like when you're pregnant but not showing, ya know.... you never forget that you're pregnant, just like I never forget I have Lupus (except for those short blips in time that I feel ok). But no one knows because it doesn't show. And I want to scream "Why are you asking me to do that? Don't you know/understand I have Lupus? I can't do that." And then I feel like I'm being such a cop out.

Vickie G

One More Time

Our beautiful, wonderful Mary Mike got me to thinking with her comment about how we go through pain, fatigue, surgeries, new medications, new doctors, new tests, etc. time and time again so that I put a little something together that we all can relate to (or, maybe I was having an out of body experience, and this won't make any sense to anyone and maybe even me if I read it again, but here goes)

If I hear how good I look "one more time" I will try very hard to smile and say thank you.

If you get upset with me "one more time" for canceling plans at the last minute, will you understand and forgive me?

If we change my meds "one more time" and I have a bad reaction does anyone care that I've just wasted more money I don't have on something I can't use?

If I tell you "one more time" that I'm in so much pain that even my hair hurts, will you understand or just think I'm being a drama queen?

When I tell you that I am so very tired and weak, can you just, "one more time" fend for yourself?

When my arms don't have the strength "one more time" to put away the groceries after shopping, do you think I'm just being a wimp?

When my legs give out on the stairs "one more time" will God be there to catch me before I break my neck? (So far, I've been able to catch myself, but that is one of my biggest fears,...well, that and drowning.)

When my neck and shoulders hurt like I'm carrying the weight of the world, will I be able to handle the stress, "one more time"?

When, "one more time", I'm having one of my sad days, will you really
understand my tears?

When, "one more time" I feel like giving up, will you encourage me to go on?

When I'm frustrated, "one more time", about how I look, will you tell me I'm still beautiful (not that I ever was, LOL)?

When I nod off "one more time" while we're watching a movie, will you tell me what I missed?

When I can't remember "one more time" where I put something or what someone said, can we just laugh about it?

How many "one more times" will there be when I can't button my shirt or wear a favorite necklace, or pick up my grandchild or just do what normal people can...

So that's the mystery of Lupus. Lupus is a puzzle of life, and we just have to make the pieces fit as best we can.

But, aside from all of this, there will always be "one more time" that we'll be able to count on our wonderful Lupies family for the support and understanding we need.

Georgia

Hello, "New"

You are NOT ALONE! There are so many of us out there. We are a group of people who are hidden because we feel too lousy to get out and make any noise about this disease. I too, have suffered for many years. Somehow I made it through raising 3 children with all the terrible symptoms of Lupus before a doctor finally ran some test and said "oooppsss" you have Lupus. Unfortunately, my diagnosis came so late in the disease that I haven't been able to get it under control. I am saddened that you have this disease, but encouraged that you have an early diagnosis and hopefully you will find an aggressive treatment plan.

I had a friend tell me that I bring my bad days upon myself because I spend too much time in bed or resting. Ok, that helps... Or how about this one... I read a popular positive religious leader's book on how to make your life better. His basic premise is that I have allowed the disease into my life because I haven't expected to be cured....I am a victim of this disease because I haven't claimed victory over it... Trust me, I have tried to ignore this disease, tried to live like I was imagining it, prayed for healing, forgiveness, and better days, written in my "grateful" journal, played positive music, read encouraging books, hung around positive people, etc.

I do think these things help, but they haven't cured me. There isn't a cure, only ways to accommodate the disease. I pray that my cocktail of medications will someday help me go into remission or at the very least, help me make it through my most painful days and tolerate all the other plagues that come with Lupus. So, to sum things up, you are not alone; yes, people are probably looking, but maybe, just maybe, they are thinking, "What a brave woman." If not, that's what you can imagine they are thinking.

Good luck and know that I am here in cyber land thinking of you. I know your pain and I care about you and your struggles. Stay strong and take care of you.

Beth

Comments by Others:

Here are some of the comments made to me by people when I told them I have Lupus:

1. You have Lupus? When are you going to die?
2. Why aren't you at home in bed so you can get better? If you rest it will get better within a couple of days.
3. Stay away from me; I don't want to get it.
4. Lupus isn't a real illness.
5. I had Lupus once; it went away in a week
6 You're fine; there is nothing wrong with you. The doctors are dumb.
7. Did you get it from having sex with someone?
8. Did you tell your kids that you are going to die soon?
9. Maybe I caught it from you; I 've had a sore throat for two days!

Susan Myrick

About Faith:

Oh Jane I am so sorry for the spiritual condemnation you have been put under. I remember the 'claim and gain' when I had prayer for migraines. The next morning I had my head in the toilet bowl, dry heaving because there was nothing left to up chuck. My husband came in and said, "I'll take you to emerg for a shot." I said, "Ulgggh no, I am okay. I - ulgggh I don't have a migraine ulgggh (dry heaving) I am healed."

I have learned more from the suffering than from being healed. I have learned to forgive, to be tolerant of others misunderstandings and trust even when not understanding the whys of suffering. My sister had prayer for her vision then she drove without her 'visuals' Thank God someone wasn't harmed.

Our son Chuck has had 18 years of miracles that even the nephrologist has recorded. I guess it all sums up to that we are not God. What doesn't break us - makes us who we are. Jane, guess what? We found this group. I am so computer brain dead, that for me, this is a miracle.

Be well and welcome to the Lupies
Val

Susan Myrick's Story

I want to tell you my story of survival. Many people find out they have an illness and they give up. I have lived my life as a survivor. When I was born my parents were told to take me home and love me because I would not live to be two weeks old. As time went and I survived, my parents were told that if I could survive to be five years old and weigh 25 pounds the doctors would be able to attempt open-heart surgery.

I had ASD, which is a hole between the two upper chambers. This can now be repaired without surgery, but in 1964 it was all an experiment. My prognosis was not good. Open-heart surgery in the early 1960's was still experimental. At age five and at barely 25 pounds, the day came for my surgery. My family was told that it would take a miracle for me to survive. I can remember the doctors drawing on my chest to decide how they should make the cut. In the end they tried a new cut for cosmetic purposes so I could wear a bikini. The surgery was successful but once again my family was not given hope. They were told I would never live to be 30 and there was no way I would have any children. I am now 50 have three children and three grandchildren. I also work a full time job.

I started having migraines at age 17. As the years went by I found that I tired very easily. The doctors ignored my complaints. They told me I was a new mother and it was normal to be tired. When I reached my mid 30's I started experiencing achy joints and strange rashes on my legs and chest. I was told the rashes were stress and dry skin. The achiness was ignored. Eventually I was told I had Fibromyalgia and there was nothing that could be done. Over the years I was hospitalized multiple times, each time being made to feel that I was crazy. I was told I needed therapy. I went to see a couple of different therapists and they also said I needed intense therapy.

As the years went by my family also thought it was all in my head. They felt I was looking for attention and that there was nothing wrong with me. The first time Lupus was suggested to me, my primary care said she thought that Lupus was a possibility and sent me to a rheumatologist. He barely examined me and gave me a shot of cortisone, to help the pain in my hip. After many more hospitalizations and after spending a week in intensive care after a stroke, my symptoms continued to get worse. There were days when I couldn't walk and I could barely get out of bed. I was in the emergency room multiple times. During one of these visits a team of doctors suggested Lupus again. At this time I had a new primary care doctor. She had a nurse practitioner that listened to my story and for the first time in many years I was told that I was not crazy and that I had a real illness. She then ordered multiple tests and told me about a rheumatologist she wanted me to see. When she got the results back they pointed towards Lupus but she did not confirm anything. She wanted to wait for the rheumatologist. When I first saw him I was scared and hopeful. He ordered many more tests and told me he would see me when he had the results. He listened to me and was very sympathetic but would not speculate on what was wrong with me. When all of the results were in, he saw me and confirmed that I have Lupus.

This was in September 2007 after many years of not knowing. I always knew something was wrong. I had mixed emotions. Fear of the unknown and joy to put a name to my illness. At first I gave in to the illness but I have learned that I can't give in to it and my family has learned to accept that Mom is ill and that I can't always do everything. Often people look at me and can't understand why I take an elevator instead of stairs or why sometimes I move so slowly. I am on multiple medications with many unpleasant side effects, none of which are specific for Lupus. I find that scary!

Diagnosis to Change
Val Owen Carlson's Story

The diagnosis wasn't the best news of the week. I looked at Dr. Chan and matter of factly replied, "So I guess I am hooped."

I drove slowly home, wondering how many more times I would be able to drive past the Thrift shop, the Bargain store, the Seniors' Home, the dear neighbor who has all the novelty woodwork in his yard, Eleanor and Clayton who wave, rain or shine, as we drive down our street towards home.

The ordinary mundane drive home became a series of events that suddenly became an appreciation for familiarity and stability that remain consistent no matter what the diagnosis. I began looking at other daily incidences with a new appreciation.

Something changed in my heart even though the surroundings were the same with the dreariness of the beginning of spring prior to the trees budding, the dirty snow in the ditches, the sludge before the newness of life and hope. Wow! Just as I was going through a season of adjustment. Suddenly, I realized that before I die I am going to Live!

No one has insight into how many days we have on this earth. Each day is a gift and it is up to us, to make the most of it. Do we waste precious time on conversations that are idle or shred another's self esteem? The Bible says that, 'What we say with our words can go forth as either a curse or a blessing.' I made it my goal to speak forth encouragement and blessing. To let go of the things that weigh me down with negative feelings and attitudes that do not edify but condemn and hinder another while at the same time rob myself of peace and joy.

So 'this is the first day of the rest of my life' and like everyone, I do not know when my last day on earth will be .... but I do know that I will live each day that I have to the fullest, knowing that one day, I will stand before my Creator and I will have to answer for the words spoken to and about others.

I will answer for how I lived with a life sentence of having Lupus but not allowing Lupus to have me. I choose to do what I can to the best of my abilities for the day and be thankful that sundown means that the sun will come up again and a new day will bring new opportunities, and I will do what I can and not worry about what I can't.

It is not too late to have a new season of adjustment and begin anew to speak words of encouragement to those around you, in your little corner of our world. You can be the instrument to speak encouragement. Your words can speak hope to someone who wakes in hopelessness and shuts their eyes at the end of day in that same state of mind and emotions. Right here, right where you are, you can make a huge difference in someone's life, no matter what the diagnosis.

Misdiagnosis
Shirley Day's Story

My present age is 49. The last 18 years, I have had SLE, which I had never heard of until 1992 when I was diagnosed, although the symptoms started a lot earlier. The first problem was spontaneous bruising followed by pains in the joints, feeling generally unwell and very fatigued.

It all started in 1978 when I began to suffer from abdominal pains and nausea. This went on for a quite a length of time. I underwent several tests at the hospital but nothing was ever found. In the end, the doctors decided it was a psychological problem and discharged me.

After this I never felt completely well. I also remember developing a strange rash across my face and on my nose , I never went to the doctors with this as they had already labeled me as having a psychological problem. Instead, I purchased a very good make up to conceal the rash; unfortunately by then my health was getting worse. I tried to live a normal life but never felt completely well.

Then one night I was at a friends party and I blacked out and dropped to the floor. I thought this could have been due to the heat. After this, I blacked out three times in the space of two months. I went to see my GP who informed me that "women have a tendency to faint. These are typical fainting attacks and no suggestion of epilepsy." He also stated it could have been a psychological problem

I was discharged with no review but the problem continued. In the two year period that followed I was having intermittent black outs. I decided to go and see my doctor again in case there was an underlying problem.

This time he sent me to see a consultant from the hospital. He thinks the problems are related to anxiety but is also a little worried that they could be petit mal attacks and would therefore arrange for an EEG with a review. When he obtained the results, I found a letter to the neurophysiologist.

He asks can you please perform an EEG on this young girl who had had a two-year history of intermittent fainting attacks but she doesn't have fits. I am wondering whether they are petit mal attacks and would there value an EEG.

The consultant reassured me that although I had borderline epilepsy it could be controlled by medication. Previous to this appointment I had lost my job because the blackouts were upsetting and frightening my work colleagues. I had just been informed I had borderline epilepsy, now in the letter to my gp he states *the patient's EEG is abnormal but not diagnostic of epilepsy. I note you have started her on tegretol 100mgs to be taken 4 times daily which were stopped prior to EEG, I have spoken to patient and mum about epilepsy and fits and I have also reassured her these are very minor and can be controlled. I would like to review in 4 months time unless there is a problem.*

The number of attacks was increasing. The consultant told me there were no neurological signs but he also increased my tegretol for 200mgs to be taken four times daily. He also arranged for me to have a further EEG and the results were the same as the previous one: slight disturbance but not diagnostic of epilepsy. I was now taking 800 mgs of tegretol, having faints but no fits.

Although I was taking tegretol every day I was still passing out 5 to 10 times each day. I remember I used to feel really strange and I would get a metallic taste in my mouth. As this was getting more frequent I made yet another visit to my GP who made a phone call to the consultant to see if he could see me earlier.

It wasn't just a simple faint; apparently, I was jerking. I went back to see my GP and told him what had happened. He sent me to see the consultant again as I had actually had a fit. When I went to see the consultant he increased the epileim to 200mgs 4 times daily so I'm now taking 800mgs of epilem and 800mgs of tegretol but the problem started to get worse. I was having regular fits now, not just faints

I was feeling really ill. Apparently after one test they found I was having a toxic effect with the drugs but nothing was done. I was beginning to feel very depressed and I could not be left on my own. I had all my independence taken from me and I was housebound, also I had to be looked after like a child. During this time I had quite a few different tests done; it was also suggested by one consultant that he thought a partial lobotomy was the only way I was going to get any control of the seizures

During 1989, I was taken in as an inpatient as I was very ill with pneumonia. In fact, in the months leading up to the pneumonia I had had quite a few bouts of pleurisy. I actually got the pneumonia at Christmas time and I spent Christmas in hospital. It took me quite a while to recover from this. By this time, I was taking 1300 mgs of tegretol, 800mgs of epilim and 400mgs of phenytoin other wise known as epanutin and also a new drug called vigabatrin, which hadn't been on the market long. I was taking 3000mgs of this at the end of 1990 when I was having vast numbers of fits and also feeling suicidal. I could see no end to this suffering and pain.

I was admitted to another hospital as an inpatient. It was whilst I was in there that the consultant came to see me. He sat on the end of my bed and told me he had spoken to my parents and told them I had been wrongly diagnosed and all the seizures I had had were induced by the meds.

I was very upset and in shock. He told me to stop taking all the meds as he wanted me off them; usually they are reduced and you're weaned off, but he stopped them suddenly. After a few months of being drug free I started to feel very unwell and fatigued and I was also bruising spontaneously. This was what led up to me being diagnosed with Lupus.

I had never heard of Lupus until then. I did start legal proceedings after being told I was epileptic but I didn't get anywhere. I fought the case for 9 years.

Labels:

Robin,

I am now 61 years old, was called everything from "lazy to sinfully lazy" as a young girl and young woman. I worked from the age of ten, and had to retire from active employment at the grand old age of 47. The doctors are STILL debating about my having Lupus, in spite of being successfully treated with Plaquenil for over thirty years, in spite of test results which are all over the map, in spite of heart, kidney, and central nervous system involvement, and countless medical incarcerations. Yeah, I am just "sinfully lazy". Uh-huh.

Labels hurt, and even more, they can kill. Just one prejudiced doctor can make life a living hell for us because all he/she sees is someone who doesn't move around much, or has weight issues due to several autoimmune disorders and the treatments used to "fix" them. I have run the gamut, but I refuse to let idiots rule my life. I demand quality care, and I make so much noise right out in front of God and everybody, they are embarrassed into doing something.

Hey, it's your life we're talking about, here, and if you want to keep it and some semblance of enjoyment in it, you have to make noise. Just my take on living life in the Lupus Lane. Loving hugs, MM

Butterflies and Doctors and Wolves, Oh My!"
Donna

Hi, Val,

I was really shocked when my doctor told me I had Lupus. I had been having increased mouth sores and this incredible exhaustion. I had to keep canceling stuff, mostly with my parents, and they couldn't understand why I couldn't just get up, get in the car, and drive. I was doing good to walk to the bathroom. And on top of all of this, I had this pain that wouldn't go away. My PCP wouldn't give me any pain meds, and wouldn't refill my Tramadol or my Celebrex.

I was literally thrown to the wolves. I had several appointments with my GI. I had been having bouts of pancreatitis, and had to have an emergency gall bladder surgery which landed me on a vent for 24 hours.

A few months before, with my first bout, they came in my room, and I had stopped breathing. I had almost died twice, and my PCP didn't care. She wouldn't even get copies of my hospital records or anything. She was more concerned with the weight I was putting on.

I finally called a rheumy who took my insurance, and that was the absolute best thing I had done in months. He dx'ed my fibro which made sense for the pain.

There wasn't a muscle or joint that didn't hurt. He took blood tests, and made a follow up appointment, and its that visit that I was dx with Lupus and Sjogren's.

I am a retired RN and never saw the wolf coming. My parents didn't take my dx seriously, just like they didn't take me being on a vent seriously. they didn't even visit me. My dad had an employee that had Lupus, and he said that she died of something other than Lupus. We all know that that isn't true.

My mother's family all died of lung diseases before they were 50, and my younger sister died in Feb of strokes. My PCP takes my HTN non-seriously, and that really bothers me. It doesn't bother me to think about the end of my life...considering family history, I will probably be very glad to see it come.

Only those who have Lupus understand fully what we go through. I am so glad to have found this group, and a friend like you, Val. I feel that if we were closer, we would be great friends.

One of the only things that is getting me down now is my back. I also have 7 bulging disks that are really starting to bother me. I am planning to start a diet after New Year's. and have a lot to lose, but I have more to lose if I don't. I am not a candidate for bariatric surgery due to my proneness to pancreatitis. Please remember me in your prayers, Val. I really need the strength to lose this weight.

Much love and many hugs to my Canuck sister!
Vicki

Coping:
Vicki,

I have been a groupie lupie since Sept. so I am still a newbie. At first I was so grateful and excited about finding a support group. I read every post and was in awe that I was normal after all (some may beg to differ) and then reality hit. Lupus is real and it doesn't have to have a definite diagnosis, the symptoms speak where the Drs' don't. Lupus.

I was overwhelmed and afraid of the Wolf. There are many frustrations, no mores and unable tos, even if you could. We begin to weigh things out carefully. i.e. if I do this.... I won't be able to do that later. Commitments can't always be met so you just do the best you can AND THAT IS OK because like Doris Christine wrote, you want to be here ten years. from now. You stop trying to explain to people because we don't look sick so our reasons look more like excuses. You learn to smile and say, I don't care (about trivial things you can't change anyway) you learn to 'not sweat the small stuff' so in some ways because of Lupus we learn lessons that some never learn. Lupus seems to have a way of taking the striving out of us and that is good. Our priorities become focused and that too is good. Hopefully we will become better and not bitter and more aware of others around us who are struggling.. .....it doesn't have to be Lupus Vicki, everyone has struggles of some kind. The good news is that we have each other to cheer us on, we are not alone and it will be OK.

You will be OK, Vicki, and three months from now you will be writing to encourage a new kid on the block who is scared, frustrated and relieved to know that they are not on this journey alone.

Be well,
Val

Pain and Other Symptoms:

Julie:

I am so sorry you are having this problem. It is so frustrating to have a significant symptom that can't be seen, felt, or heard by a physician. It doesn't mean it doesn't exist and you didn't use up your wine factor with your physician when you talk about it.

Symptoms are an important part of knowing how your Lupus is at the moment. Unfortunately, some symptoms stay with you for years or even life, but some symptoms fade in and out and you just learn how to deal with each.

I have had what my family calls my "stupid leg" for years. At times I have to physically lift it up and down to get in or out of a chair or bed. I can be walking fine one minute and it will start dragging the next. Sometimes I think it lives in its own zip code and acts like a teenager that doesn't want to comply with the rules of the house.

This happens more when I am tired or stressed. Sometimes my whole leg aches, sometimes just my knee. I have had an x-ray, MRI, nerve conduction test, and every blood test know to man. I have been seen by many doctors including a neurologist and a doctor who only works with feet, knees, ankles, and legs. The tests always come back negative or inconclusive and the doctors are always perplexed.

The only test I haven't had is a spinal tap and I just can't get my mind wrapped around someone sticking a needle in my spine while I am awake, so I have passed on that one.

Continue to whine and complain...symptoms are important even if the problem doesn't have a solution, maybe yours will. Hope someone helps you soon

Beth

And the saga continues.... Another hospitalization and trial by fire

Dear Lupie Friends,

If your memory is anything like mine, you need a little refresher course in what has been happening with me. Since the third week of November I have been battling pericarditis. My rheumatologist has played the "it's just Lupus and you will get through this, just take Vicodin until it stops hurting" card which has infuriated my cardiologist.

The two doctors have had several phone calls that were heated exchanges of how my condition should be treated medically. The first of Jan, I was still in bed feeling like I was having a heart attack every time the pain meds wore off. My cardio talked my rheumy into a hospitalization that resulted in 500 mg of IV steroids.

He never came to the hospital. I was out of pain when I left the hospital, but the fatigue was unbearable. As the week progressed, the pain began to return. Last Wednesday, I dragged myself out of bed and drove myself 90 miles to an appointment with my endocrinologist (which has been scheduled for 6 months and impossible to change).

He came into the exam room with the gloom and doom face and told me that my body is not absorbing the synthroid and my numbers were off. I had my thyroid removed, so my body doesn't have a backup plan. He asked me if I was having fatigue problems... you think?

Anyway, before I could tell him my pericarditis saga he was already listening to my heart. He gave me some breathing commands and stepped back with a look of terror on his face and told me that I needed to go to the ER because I had a severe pericardial rub.

I told him that my cardiologist's office was right down the street, so I would call her office and tell her what was going on, which he made me do while I was still in the exam room. The lovely little girl that answers the phone quickly told me that they didn't have any room to squeeze me in. I explained the problem and told her to get the message to the dr ASAP because it was an emergency. She said she would call me right back.

REALLY? Two hours later, I was sitting in a Starbucks still waiting, unmedicated and hurting. I finally had enough and drove to the office and walked in just as the cardio entered the front desk area. She took one look at me and yelled for her nurse to come get me in a room.

(Needless to say, she hadn't been given the message.)

Long story short...I had another EKG and sonogram and now the lining of my heart is thickening and inflamed. Again, she called my rheumy (who still hadn't found the time to see me since my last hospital stay) and he told her he could see me sometime next week. OMG!!!! She lost it and had to leave the room to regain her composure.

When she came back in this is what she said, "I have fired your rheumatologist and arranged for you to see another one after you spend two days in the hospital. You should never tolerate a dr who is too busy to see you or talk to you especially with other doctors listing your condition as life threatening. If you disagree with this you need to find another cardiologist. I can't stand to see you treated without regard to your pain and suffering. I can't treat your Lupus; I can only treat the damage it causes to your heart.

"The damage it is causing now is preventable if treated NOW. If not, you are looking at open-heart surgery and life long consequences. " Well, she convinced me. I drove myself to the hospital and called my husband, who was 90 miles away at work, and was admitted.

I was released two days later to go to the new rheumatologist office. The experience was positive from the moment we entered the office. My husband and I were met with smiles and compassion. We were seen 10 minutes before the scheduled time, the rheumy spent 45 minutes in the room and actually read my typed and dated symptoms and treatments 1 page outline of how the disease has progressed and when medications were added and subtracted along with the last four lab results.

He told me how impressed he was that I had such detailed information and how much time it would save him. He did a complete exam and asked us if we wanted a second opinion or wanted to change doctors. My husband told him that we have been playing the "doctor shuffle" and that the only doctor pushing for my well being has been my cardiologist and we were looking for a doctor who was willing to take control of my total care and get t me back on track.

This doctor looked my husband in the eyes and told him that he would love to take my case and be in charge. He said my Lupus is out of control because my treatment is too conservative and he wants to hit it hard and fast. He explained that my heart was not the only organ involved. The blood test suggest that my kidneys are compromised and the ultrasound performed in the hospital shows that I have a non alcoholic fatty liver that needs to be treated.

I told him I haven't been told any of that and I only know that I feel like dog pooh most of the time and I'm tired of feeling this way. He told us he was ready to get me to a better place and said let start by emptying your prescription bag out and going over each one...WOW!

The rest of the time he spent talking us through his plan of action. We left with his promise of being an active physician and with the feeling of hope for the first time in 3 years.

I go back to the cardio on Friday and then they are going to talk about starting on his new plan of action.

I so hope this is the start of a better life for me.
Beth

You Know You're a Lupie When...

"

You go inside, pay for $10.00 worth of gas, get back in your car and drive off.... without pumping the gas.
After doing that a couple of times...(feeling like I just made a cash donation to one of the oil companies!) I now put the hose in the gas tank BEFORE I pay for the gas. (But then I could pull another Lupie trick and drive off with the hose still in the gas tank....) LOL!
Marilyn

You know you are a lupie when"

"You turn on the burner, set the skillet on it, and when the smoke alarms go off, you wonder. Why are the alarms going off...I forgot my skillet!! Vicki in Texas (this happened last week)

You know you are a lupie when...

You get poked for blood 8 times because you are so swollen before they finally get a trace of blood for your lab work

You know you are a lupie when...
You spell cash as *chash*
Robyn

You know you are a lupie when........ You talk to someone, forget you talked to them. So you tell them again to talk about what you just talked about but can't remember. Stef

You know you are a lupie when...

You let the dog out to do her business, and then later on in the day get surprised when you find her shivering on the porch when you go out to dump the trash. Poor baby.

MM

You Know You're a Lupie when:

The telephone rings, and you pick up the TV remote to answer...

Marilyn

You know you are a lupie when...

You...........sheesh! I forgot! Val

Coping and Depression

Each case of Lupus is unique in appearance, timing, intensity, and personal impact on the patient. This is just how the disease works on each of us. One person has intensely painful episodes of disease activity that affects certain parts of their body, while another person with similar symptoms will have completely different areas of their body affected, and perhaps for much longer periods of time. As I said, it is unique to the individual.

First thing you need to do is become proactive in your own case. Read the articles in the FILES link on our home page, and ask your doctor pointed questions. Don't take "we will have to wait and see" for an answer, and ask about specific pain meds to keep you comfortable while you wait for Plaquenil or other drugs to do their work. Remember that Lupus is a PROGRESSIVE disease that waxes and wanes, but is always moving along.

You are not in control of it, but you ARE in control of your attitude toward your illness. You CAN control your life to the extent that you CAN develop a sense of humor in spite of painful days, you CAN come to the group as you did today for comfort, information, and hope, and you CAN be treated with antidepressants to help you control your sadness and avoid despair when your disease flares. It may be necessary to try several of them to find one that works well for you, but you should know that Clinical Depression is part and parcel of living with Lupus and many other major diseases. It is not a temporary problem and needs to be treated as soon as possible. It can make all the difference in how you cope with Lupus.

I don't want to overwhelm you, but this is information you need to know. Hope it is helpful.

Loving hugs,
MM

Lupus Poem

Invisible Scourge
by Margaret (Beth) Lindsley 5/20/09

Hidden behind the smile
Evident by movement
Guttural sounds by day
And whimpering by night

Determination and pride
Mixed with hopelessness
Trapped within dreams
Of normality

Measuring time by appointments
Fearing the next poke and prod
Noticing friends disconnecting
While family acclimates

Planning nutrition around pills
Clothing by comfort
Activity by pain
Makeup by tears

Questions run rampant
Invited? Uninvited? Guest? Resident?
Answers evade understanding
Fighting takes its toll

Pain and Lupus and Doctors:

Dear Tigger,

I understand your frustration with the neuros. Mine drives me crazy. She says "hmmmm" a lot and runs lots of tests and then doesn't tell me anything. I only see her reports when I ask my rheumy what she reported. She always lists depression as the #1 diagnosis. UGH! REALLY? You think?

If she hurt this bad she would be depressed too...or how about this...figure out why I have pain and eliminate it and maybe I won't be depressed. She always makes me feel like I overemphasize my gait problems. I find it quite embarrassing that I trip and fall in public and sometimes can't lift my leg up enough to get out of a car or climb stairs and I think that is a big problem at 48.

About the fibro pain part...we all have different levels of pain because of the difference in pain receptors. Go figure, I didn't go to medical school but I know better than to say something so stupid to a patient in pain. How does someone explain the pain we feel? My dr always makes me circle a number from 1-10 describing my pain level that day. I think that is wrong. Today might be a 6 and tomorrow might be a 10. I never circle anything and he always gets irritated and asks me questions and then he picks a number. Hahahaha...I make him do his job...you know...talk to me.

EEEKKK. I didn't know I was so irritable this morning, but reading what you have gone through just sends me spiraling through the past 3 years of this horrible journey. Frustrating, exhausting, depressing, and isolating.

You are right...some drs are idiots. Ok, I am going to try some yoga and calm myself back down.

I am here with you,

Beth

What is With the Dark Hole??????

Angela,

We can likely all relate to the dark hole. I will do whatever I can to stay out of there, it was so bad. There is a fable about a donkey who was thrown into a deep dry well and the owner was shoveling dirt into the hole in an attempt to bury the old donkey.

The donkey shook the dirt off his back and tramped it down, same thing with the next shovel full. Just shook it off. Eventually the donkey could see daylight and he was able to step out of the hole. The donkey didn't give in to all the dirt being thrown on him.

You will see daylight, Angela. Don't despair. Soon you will be posting someone who thinks they are all alone in a black hole but you will be able to encourage them that you have been there done it and there is always hope. Hang on, sweetie. You have many who are praying for you. And sending a hand to help you out.

Love and prayers,
Val

What is With the Dark Hole??????

Angela, sweetie,

I had to jump out of my "ketchup" mode and get to you pronto!! Please, please know that although we're on anti depressants we still get times when we feel like you but if you've been in this dark hole for a while you really need to call the doctor. You may need an increase in the Lexapro or something different. If you read the info that comes with anti depressant meds, they all say that a side effect can be depression and thoughts of suicide which I always thought was a misprint...anti depressant causing depression.. .what gives but it's true it can happen. I want you to concentrate on your wonderful e mail handle of pleasure hope and joy and know that you are worthwhile and as one of God's children, you do serve a very special purpose. If you still feel like this tomorrow, call the doctor!!! Georgia

Heat and Sun, etc

Robyn,

Last year my husband drove me 13 hours to see my son in New Mexico. The day after I arrived I went into a major flare so I called my rheumy to tell him I was out of town and needed help. He told me that the sun I received through the windows in the car wasn't any different than standing out side. Duh! I didn't even think about it that way.

The sun wasn't on me so I didn't think I was being exposed. Now, I am officially a vampire. If I venture out during the day I take every precaution possible. I am now considered "the woman in the hat" and was even asked recently why I always cover up my body even when it is 90+ degrees outside. I personally think that is a rude question, so I just smiled and said, "because I like this outfit" I mean, what was I supposed to say? No one wants to hear my Lupus saga.

Here's to being a vampire and living life in the lupie lane.
Beth

Mouth and Lip Sores

"   I have had mouth sores and lips sores chronically for about 15 years.

I have had sores in my mouth that hurt so bad I curled up in a fetal position and cried for days at a time. I asked the rheumy and my internist for help and neither knew anything to do except salt water or hydrogen peroxide.

My dentist gave me prescription for something called Pink Magic. The directions said to swish a tablespoon of the liquid around in my mouth, so I fell for it. My tongue began swelling and I had a panic attack that triggered a seizure...good stuff huh?

I finally figured out that if I used a q-tip on the blister it helped with the pain without causing me to cut off my oxygen supply. Unfortunately, it did nothing to speed the recovery process, but it did work long enough for me to be able to eat. The good news is that since I've been on imuran for the past six months, I have had very few mouth sores and they have been minor and healed quickly. Not sure if this is a coincidence or the imuran. All I know is that mouth sores stink!
Beth

Vicki:
Cut that out! I mean about seeing yourself in a wheelchair in the next few years. It's okay to be absolutely furious that you have Lupus, and yell and punch pillows all you want. But don't give in to it. Don't let it win. If you see yourself debilitated, you might just be that way. But we don't know the future, and especially with Lupus being the way it is.... unpredictable.

I'm not being pollyanna-ish about this, like "think good thoughts," etc. but just being stubborn that I'm in charge, not this illness.

Oh, and yes, I'm aware that the discs may cause you some mobility problems in the future, but I think the doctors have more success with those issues than with Lupus. At least surgeons can go in and take out stuff that's causing trouble, or patch things, etc. Don't we wish they could do the same with Lupus?

I can see it all now: "Dr. McDreamy please report to OR2 for a Lupusectomy. "

Marilyn

Telling Your Family

Terrie,

It's important to remember that healthy people will never understand chronic illness. In their estimation, you should be able to just "get over it." Yeah, right. It isn't ever going to go completely away, and it will take Plaquenil some weeks to months to fully kick in and do its job.

Also, I began with pain and fatigue, dx'd with RA, then with skin lesions, and then with SLE. It took UC San Francisco teaching hospital doing multiple tests on me for years to get a dx of SLE, and even then, they called it "Lupus Suspect", not SLE.

I didn't get the "suspect" removed until nearly five years ago. I was dx'd at thirty, and am now sixty. This disease process is one for the books, and I would tell your family that 80% of DLE (skin Lupus) patients develop Systemic Lupus Erythematosus within ten years of the skin dx. That pain, fatigue and complications can go with it all during the time between skin onset and system onset.

Each Lupus patient is unique. We may have the same disease, even similar symptoms, but appearance, timing, onset, intensity, variety, and which organ (the skin being the largest organ in the body) is attacked, is unique to each patient. This is why Lupus is so difficult to diagnose (dx) and to treat effectively.

Tell your family that your body will dictate, from now on, what you can and cannot do, for how long, and how often. That, if you do not listen to and accommodate your body, you WILL end up sicker and possibly going to the ER. We know this because we have experienced it for ourselves.

It isn't in our heads, or caused by being too emotional, it IS a real disease process, is NOT curable, and only temporary relief from symptoms is ever achieved. I have had three long remissions in my life, but in the last ten years, even short remissions are rarities. I have had symptoms since I was 12 years old, and prior to that had Thyroid problems, too, from age five.

Also, if you have children, the odds of them developing this disease, or another autoimmune problem, is much greater, than for those children whose parents do not have autoimmune issues. We have many members who are just now having their children tested due to familiar symptom patterns.

So, honey, don't let your family try to put you in denial, or allow them to disbelieve your situation. Feel free to print a copy of this email and give it to them. They need to step up. Period.

Loving hugs,
MM

Doctor Visits:

Dear Daisy,

I am so sorry about your first visit. I too, had a terrible first visit with my first rheumy. She discounted all of my complaints and asked me if I had Googled "Lupus" and asked if I "really" had all the symptoms I had written on the 10 tons of paperwork. Then she opened the exam door and screamed down the hallway for "a fat person to come into exam room 2" and seconds later a portly man slid into the room.

She grabbed his hands and told me to feel his joints and then had me feel my own hands. And then asked me to tell her the difference. I was speechless! I am 5'5" and weighed all of 100 pounds. What was I supposed to say? I just muttered something about my knuckles looked red and his didn't. She then asked me why I came to her office and didn't I know Lupus was a "black" disease and that I was white so the odds were I had arthritis and not Lupus AND that I just wanted to be labeled disabled and she didn't do that.

OMG! I lost it! Somewhere through my tearful tirade I told her that I had made a mistake in coming there and I wouldn't be back. She tried to calm me down and asked me if I had considered counseling? WHAT? She needed counseling and a course on how to talk to people without being a prejudiced pig!

She filled out several prescriptions and sent me for x-rays. I left defeated. My husband talked me into filling the prescriptions and getting the x-rays and was convinced that I had misunderstood her comments or just being dramatic. He promised to attend my next appointment to be a moderator.

Two months later we went back and the x-rays showed inflammation, but no evidence of arthritis. She told us that she disagreed with the radiologist report and said I had "rupus" and I could expect a five-year lifespan. She also told me that no one knew how to treat what I had and the medications were used off label, toxic, rarely worked and my life would never be the same again, so I just needed to enjoy what time and ability I had left.

My husband stood up, told her in no uncertain terms that she was a jerk and we never went back! My next-door neighbor noticed that I stopped doing my gardening and outdoor activities and came to check on me. I cried buckets of tears as I explained what I was going through.

She, too, had Lupus and I didn't even know it. She gave me her rheumy's number and told me he was wonderful. It took me a while to get the courage to call his office only to be told that they had a 4-month waiting list for new patients. I told her about the wait and she called the doctor's office and somehow got me in within the week.

Thank goodness, he is wonderful and has worked so hard to help me negotiate this beast of a disease. He has filled out tons of disability paperwork and spent much time explaining what is going on with my body. He makes me research any medications that he is contemplating so I am ready for questions before each visit. I thank my lucky stars that he is in my life. I hope that there is another doctor like him in your area. Unfortunately, sometimes you have to go through a few frogs to find a prince.   Beth

"Why is Everything So Negative?" A Question from a Visitor to the Group Who Wants us to "Just Think Good Thoughts."

Nellie,

I am so glad that you have found life on the sunny side of the street. I try my hardest to live on the same side you are on...but,(get ready for some negative)... some days I use all of my energy on trying to hide the pain I am in and need a place to vent.

Well, Nellie, this is the place. We don't mean to be negative. We hurt, we are tired, we are misunderstood, we are emotionally drained, physically spent, and most of us are dealing with major health problems that could turn deadly if we don't pay attention to our bodies.

I personally take eleven medications that remind me how sick I am. Acknowledging the facts of this terrible disease with others who are in the same boat is not negative. It keeps me sane, gives me guidance, and guess what...sometimes I even gain a sense of hope because I know that someone out there in cyber land cares about my fight against this beast.

Trust me, I make the best out of every day, only some days my best is better than other days. To tell you the truth your comment today devastated me, and turned a fairly good day into a negative one. I face comments like yours continually in my real world of people who don't understand.

I wish upon a million stars that always being positive would cure me. I am who I am. I post when I have good days, I post when I have bad days. Next time you read a post from me where I am being negative, don't read it. Wait awhile and I'll blog about something I did that I couldn't do last week. Today's not one of those days.

Sorry,
Beth

Doctors Again:

The rheumatologist was the one who decided he was looking at rosacea. So my next step is to tell them fine, send me to dermatology. .. and then neurology too, because rosacea and osteoarthritis doesn't explain my cognitive impairment. The last time I checked, rosacea doesn't cause memory loss.

Learn to live with your symptoms? You already do - that's what you tell them. I already do... now give me an understanding of WHY so I can figure out how to live my life better with them!

I'm in the same boat of wait for more symptoms. I guess they haven't yet decided that Lupus is one of those early detection for a better prognosis diseases. They're always hounding me to get other things checked, so I thought they'd be happy I brought a concern up readily. Not.

Oh, and I completely get what you're saying about wishing something serious would happen so they could pinpoint it. That sounds crazy unless you're in our shoes, right? The evening that I sat checking my provider's website over and over for my lab results on dsDNA and Anti-smith, I wished it had just shown up positive so they would actually think they had to DO something for me. A *negative test result doesn't make me healthy*. They sure seem to think it does.

As I'm telling them.. I'm not looking for a comforting diagnosis, I'm looking for an accurate one. It isn't like I'm going to be shocked. I've been prepared for the possibility, even probability that it's Lupus since before I went to ask the Dr. to run the tests.

I hope you get better answers soon.

Tala

Well, Crapolie, Anyway!

Oh, Val.

What an idiot that man is. With the symptoms you reeled off, it's obvious to anyone -- even a doctor! -- That you have Lupus. Classic Lupus. No question about it.

And with vasculitis, no less. You need to be on Cytoxan or Imuran for the vasculitis. I took it for quite a while when my ankles wouldn't flex. They used to call that, "foot dropsy" and it makes it hard to walk. This is when I had to sleep in high-topped lace up tennis shoes so my ankles would be trained in their proper position for walking.

I would follow up with the hospital administrator, or Director of Medicine. The head honcho. State the reasons you are unhappy with his treatment, or non-treatment-- of you, and how dismissive he was, telling you he "has an appointment with a patient" -- like *you're* NOT a patient? Make a copy or three or four and send them to anybody who is associated with the hospital or department and even the Canadian equivalent of the County Medical Association. This man should not be practicing medicine, with his attitude and ineptitude.

And then, send a copy to his mother..... 😛

Most of all, though, take care of yourself and find a REAL physician who will take you seriously and treat you like a real person. Your general practitioner should be included in the loop, too, so he won't refer this rheumy to anyone else. And he can connect you with someone who is human.

Marilyn

Flarin' Along Like a Hurricane

Val,

Tell your hb that stomach upset, gas, bloating, runs, blockages, et al, are common in Lupies, as are unique and fascinating other physical phenomena. The Malar Rash, which can appear anywhere on the body, but is best known for its butterfly shape over the nose and cheeks (I even get antenna on my forehead! And, no, I can't contact Mars.) and can be the only color in our faces at times. Isn't this fun?

Aches, sudden spasms, sharp needling pains, all the weirdness of an ordinary Lupie day, is something no one can understand who hasn't experienced it firsthand, as we well know. I think it takes an extraordinary person to even attempt to understand it who hasn't lived it. And, I believe spouses, children, and friends who truly try to be supportive deserve an award for their efforts.

I also think we Lupies deserve an award just for surviving from day to day. It is often like living in the center of a hurricane and being occasionally sucked into the outer wall of the storm and beaten to a pulp. If we're lucky, we get thrown back into the eye of the storm to rest awhile, then we're back out in it, again.

And, we can't plan when or how we will be from one hour to the next, and we are at the mercy of the whims of Lupus.

I have observed that most of us who are surviving this disease are type A personalities, with drive, imagination, and very high pain tolerances. This damn disease gets the best of the best of us. I, for one, refuse to let it win all the time get to win one once in a while. So there!!!

Loving hugs,
MM

Kelly Greenway's Story

My name is Kelly. I am twenty-seven years old from Sydney, Australia and I was officially diagnosed with Systemic Lupus Erythematosus (SLE) when I was seventeen. The diagnosis came after I was extremely ill in my final year of high school. I contracted glandular fever but I had symptoms of SLE even before that. I was constantly fatigued; I would come home from school and sleep up until 6 p.m. and go back to sleep at 10.p.m and still feel fatigued waking up for school. As a child I wasn't well I was always in and out of hospital with asthma problems and had infections one after the other that kept me from school, but it never stopped me from smiling.

My mother and I think I was born with Lupus as I came out in a bright rash that was nothing like the eczema that developed later. Also whilst my mother was pregnant with me, my blood somehow leaked back into the umbilical cord and my mother suddenly had Anti-Nuclear Antibodies (ANA) .The doctors said it was my blood, but they weren't stressed or even worried and nobody explained to my mother what it was. At nineteen, my mother, of course, was going to trust the doctors.

At the age of eight I almost died, courtesy once again to doctors who didn't really know what they were doing. I was at my Aunt's wedding, having a great time dancing around, but early on that week I had complained about not being able to breathe properly. Mum listened to my chest but couldn't hear anything rattle like usual when I had asthma attacks. My Nan (Dad's mother) came to say goodbye; I went to kiss her goodnight when she put her hand on my forehead.

"Take her to the hospital straight away; your daughter is very sick." Well, we weren't far from the children's hospital. I was disappointed I couldn't stay and dance and talk with all the other children

The doctor looked and checked me out but instead of getting a confirmation on what was wrong with me, my mum got this: "Honestly I think your daughter is faking it." My mother hit the roof.

"How dare you accuse my daughter of something like this! She has a fever, for God's sake and you are telling me she is faking it? I want to see another doctor this minute. And I want to know who's in charge of you; they will be getting a stern letter from me."

This doctor got a colleague who listened to my chest and heard my laboured breathing; my mother also told him about the fever. He sent me straight into a ward and put me on some prednisone and a nebulizer to try and clear my chest. My mother went to get me an ice-block and when she came back I knew something was wrong, very wrong. All I could say was "Mummy, Mummy, Mummy."

I remember the drip being put in and then after that nothing, I blacked out. Turns out I had a collapsed left lung with pneumonia. I woke up in ICU not knowing how I had gotten there. I was put on medication, oxygen and plenty of bed rest. My stay in ICU was about three days before going back to the ward. They took blood tests then as well, but still no one picked up on the low white cell count.

When I was about nine I had a very bad urinary tract infection (UTI). It was so bad that I could not lift my head from a pillow and had a very high fever. The doctors at a Children's hospital suggested I was faking it; my mother was furious, I couldn't lift my head and barely speak and I was faking it?

The UTIs continued throughout my entire life, some worse than others. Sometimes I had to have trips to the E.R. to be put onto fluids and given an injection to stop the vomiting.

When I was tested again for glandular fever, I was given the all clear. I returned to school as usual until one day whilst sitting in religious studies class I suddenly felt very ill all over again. They called my mother to come and get me and I went straight back to the GP's. She immediately did some more blood tests and would ring me in the morning with the results. Until then I was to remain on bed rest. The results came back that I had glandular fever again. It's impossible to have it twice, so she knew something was up.

I had to come back into see my GP when I was feeling up to it to get tested to see if I still had glandular fever. She looked over my results and said: "That's odd, all your blood tests since you were eight have come back with a low white cell count. Have I sent you to see a hematologist?"

I was furious, although I didn't say anything impolite as much as I wanted to. Of course she made arrangements at a local hospital I was to have blood tests every week for six weeks to see what was going on with my body. After six weeks the results were in; this hematologist didn't beat around the bush. "Kelly you have something known as Systemic Lupus Erythematosus, SLE for short and some people just refer to it as Lupus. It's an autoimmune disease. I can't really tell you a lot about it because we are still discovering people have different symptoms. Tell me, do you often have urinary tract infections?" I nodded my head; I couldn't speak.

I had an autoimmune disease. What did this mean? I was seventeen and scared.

"These are also a part of Lupus, kidney problems have also been linked to Lupus. You also have something called Cyclic Neutropenia. This is where every three to four weeks your white cell count dips lower than it already is and you are more at risk of catching viruses. I will get you into see the Professor of Immunology. Now, tell me. Do you know anyone in your family that has Lupus? More often than not it's a hereditary thing." This hematologist, though, forgot to mention that I had the Anti-Nuclear Antibodies.

Some things finally clicked, like why I was sick all the time. My mother rang my father as soon as we were out of the office. My dad then piped up with, "My cousin died of that, but it was in the early 50s." I didn't say anything on the ride home. I was thinking to myself 'Great. Some old lady whom I never met but is related to me had this disease, so it's hereditary.'

When I was twenty-four I had an unplanned pregnancy. I was scared about what my mum was going to say. I was in a relationship with my current boyfriend but I wasn't married. We had discussed children many a time and I had even spoken about children with my Lupus Professor. He at one stage told me I probably would never be able to conceive children, then the next time I saw him it was if I did conceive I would probably end up miscarrying. I was really frustrated and fed up and just basically saw him for my blood work more than anything else. I didn't say anything as every time I was at his office I was always frustrated and angry or even ended up in tears. He told me at one point "We don't know that much about Lupus to tell you conclusively how it will affect you."

My pregnancy didn't go exactly as planned. I was told to come off the medication I was on for my anxiety and panic attacks as I had been taking it for so long my body was used to it and to come off it within a week was a living nightmare. I had constant headaches, and then I started getting very bad morning sickness basically from the time I found out I was pregnant. It lasted for six months and went all day and all night; I could barely keep food down. The doctors didn't seem to care, though; as long as I was hydrated, everything was fine.

I only put on two kilograms my whole pregnancy but the baby was fine and that's all that I was worried about. As the pregnancy progressed my anxiety and panic worsened. I became agoraphobic, only leaving the house for the ante-natal clinic appointments and for psychiatrist appointments. I wasn't allowed to have anything with calmative properties because it might cross the placenta. I had all day sickness for five months out of the nine

I think in total I had six ultrasounds to make sure that my baby was growing because Lupus apparently doesn't make babies grow. The baby was looking very good though and the baby's weight was on the low side but not abnormally so. I was asked at thirty weeks what kind of birth I wanted; I told them I wanted a caesarean section.

I was thirty-seven weeks pregnant, miserable from panic, anxiety, agoraphobia and having to inject myself and then this news. Once again I was sent for another scan just to make sure the baby's heart was fine. My stress levels were rising and rising and I was unaware of it. The baby's heart was looked at and the heartbeat checked and all seemed fine.

Then on the 26/6/2007 at eight a.m. my daughter, Kimberly Campbell, was born via caesarean section. I was knocked out for it all, I don't think I could stand being awake and the doctors all agreed it would be better for me and they didn't want to upset my blood pressure either as they had just gotten it under control.

I was in recovery whilst my daughter was wheeled in to meet the family: Grandmas, Great Grandmas and Daddy were all waiting. Born at only 47cm and in size 00000 clothing weighing 2.25 kilograms, we discovered later that Kimberly had a heart murmur and we were referred to see a cardiologist. Luckily for us it was discovered that the heart murmur was innocent. I was in the hospital five days after the caesarean, to keep an eye on me and make sure my Lupus didn't flare.

What the doctors neglected to tell me was that it was possible to flare anytime within the next six months.

When Kimberly was about three months of age I was going to see my Lupus specialist. I told my mum my feet hurt, almost to the point where it was so hard to walk because of the pain. We told my Lupus doctor and he checked me out saying my feet were colder than they should be but nothing unusual. The pain seemed to progress. I went to GPs who also couldn't figure it out and sent me to see other specialists; in turn these specialists couldn't find the cause, either. Kimberly was about five months old by this time and the only thing getting me through the pain was valium, two five mg tablets.

Then one day it got to the point where I couldn't even put my foot on the floor because of sheer pain; my left ankle was swollen. No one ever thought to check to see if the Lupus was flaring. My mum then decided to take me to the emergency room. I was admitted into hospital. They did test after test and sent me for a bone scan. I wasn't allowed to see my daughter on this day or the day after because of the radiation in the injection. My mood had once again gone from being happy to being very sullen and I was continuously crying from either pain or what we now think was postnatal depression.

They sent in a psychologist to see me as well as a psychiatrist to put me onto medication that would improve my mood. They then discovered that the veins and arteries in my feet are very narrow and the blood flow doesn't circulate properly. They thought about giving me surgery to open the veins thinking that may stop the pain because the blood flow would be better but then decided against it. My mum and I knew from reading things on the net that I was having a Lupus flare; all my hair was falling out in chunks, my feet hurt so badly that even turning over in a bed would cause me to cry.

I spent two months and two weeks in hospital learning to basically get over the pain and -walk again. I went back on my panic disorder medication and I felt like my old self again before the pregnancy and before the flare.

I am not on medication for Lupus. I am holding off for as long as possible. When the pain gets to be unbearable I use strong pain relief medication. Every time now that I have an infection I am always put on antibiotics. Because of the Lupus it takes me twice as long to recover than most people, even from a common cold.

I try to avoid people who are unwell with something contagious because I am likely to pick it up. My daughter is now 2 ½ years old. Last year I went to pick her up and felt something in my back just move. Turns out I slipped a disc and had sciatica because of a nerve pressing against the disc. When I went to the physiotherapist he told me "You have the tightest muscles I have seen in my nineteen years of working for this profession, more than likely due to the Lupus." Lupus struck again. Physiotherapy is like torture especially if you are already in pain.

I discovered the key to physiotherapy was taking painkillers before going so I wouldn't hurt as bad. My teeth are also affected by the Lupus, my dentist has told me.

I used to push myself in everything but now I have learned the lesson the hard way. I pace myself and am enjoying every day to the fullest. I have made a lot of friends with Lupus as well and we all share similarities; we share the good, the bad, and sometimes the humorous side of life. Lupus is a part of my life and those who surround me; some still may not understand but most have come to accept it.

Oh, Janet, that's something we all hear, all the time, from people who don't know about the devastation Lupus brings. I think Lupus is the Rodney Dangerfield of illnesses: "We don't get no respect." Some of my favorite remarks are: "Lupus? That's fatal, isn't it?" To which I reply, "Life is fatal."

And "Your depression will get lots better if you get out and walk." Heh. Getting out of bed is a real accomplishment, and they want you to suddenly spring out the door and walk?

And when I slap my Handicapped Parking card up on my windshield and get out of the car at the grocery store, some busybody always smarts off, "You're not handicapped. " Just because I'm not in a wheelchair. . Yet. To which I reply, "There are all kinds of handicaps, and one of them is ignorance."

People just don't know, and some of them actually think they're helping. One friend suggested the use of aspertame "caused" my Lupus. Well, la-ti-dah. That's kind of like being a voodoo priest telling a cancer patient they held too much anger and it turned into cancer. Sheesh.

And at least with cancer, it has a fairly predictable course of progression and treatment.   Not so with Lupus.

Welcome to our world!

Marilyn

Lupus Turns You Green?

Hi everyone,

I went to my Rheumy today and he gave me a shot of steroids right in the butt. I have been on overdrive ever since. I baked cookies for my son's class, did laundry and cleaned the house all after I got up at 4:30am. Crazy how good that stuff can make you feel.

He also doubled the dose of Quinacrine that I am on. He told me that my skin might turn darker of even a little.....wait for this ----GREEN!!!!!!!

I was like WHAT????

I am very light skinned with blond hair so I can just imagine how cute that will be. Also, my nail beds could turn blue. I am going to look like a freak!!!! LOL at least I will have a laugh watching all the people's faces when they get a look at my green skin. Hehe!

I am sure it won't be that bad. Anyway he said that my disease is not well enough controlled due to the fact that I have four kids. There is nothing I can do about that so I just have to go on more and more meds until it is controlled, I guess.

I have a question though. With the medicines that you are all on, do your symptoms go completely away or do they just get better? He gave me the impression today that they should go all the way away.

Gretchen

Green?

Gretchen,

Green sounds fun. You will have the opportunity to be the Grinch without having to dress up. You can tell everyone you are green with envy, or your green thumb has taken over your whole body, or you can tell people that you ate your money because you don't trust banks and this is a side effect, or you are a really big fan of the Green Bay Packers, or you didn't read the instructions on your pet Chia correctly and you rolled in the seeds. (Blame it on a lupie.)

Keep us posted on your greenness,
Beth

Help with Natural Pain Relief

Hi,

I want to reiterate before I go on that you need to consult with your physician before you do any of these things. Every person with Lupus has different issues. I've been going down the homeopathic road myself. My Lupus is mild so I feel like I don't want to take the strong meds (at least not yet). There are so many things online if you do searches for arthritis relief, etc

Beware for sure of immune system boosters like Echinacea. Lupus patients aren't supposed to take these. I take extra magnesium supplements for inflammation, along with ginger and tumeric. I tried Evening Primrose oil, but it didn't really do anything for me.

Castor Oil is supposed to be good as a rub in and gets deep down (warning: it's really sticky/tacky) . I've been trying that for a few days only, so I can't tell you for sure if it's really working.

You can also try essential oils such as peppermint, lavender, black pepper and eucalyptus, but make sure you don't use these on your skin straight. They must have a "carrier" oil. Olive oil or almond oil or castor oil would work.

Epsom salt is magnesium and soaking in it will help, too. Heat pads are great. I sometimes sleep with one.

Remember, not all of these will help you and PLEASE ask your doctor if you might have a condition where you shouldn't use these.

Vickie

Questions re: Lighting, Brain Fog, and Helpful vs. Unhelpful People.

Pattie,

I, too have learned to go with the flow, most of the time. I also wear a hat anywhere there is lighting that can start a headache, cause a rash, or just trigger a flare. It really helps me to remember to put on sunscreen, even on overcast days, and indoors. I still get skin lesions, but much less often by being careful about lighting, and the sun.

The brain fog really frustrates me, but I am learning to laugh at myself. My kids, on the other hand are making dark remarks about Alzheimer's. I just give them dirty looks, and when it clears up I get even. LOL

Mostly I was always so organized about the bills, appointments, etc. Now, I have to write everything down immediately or I might miss an important lab test, or double pay a bill and forget another. Drives me nuts.

As for my family, like I said, except for my two boys who are still at home, my sisters and daughter are very understanding. My doctors and business friends have learned to call me a day or so ahead of time to remind me of our appointments. And, my friends just laugh with me, and comfort me when I cry, so I am a lucky woman.

Loving hugs,
MM

Being a Survivor

Dearest Heather,

I am so very sorry. My husband left me when I had 3 small children and I was 7months pregnant. I thought my world had ended. I was only 24. I was abused physically and mentally and I didn't know what I would do ...how I would survive.

But I did. I had a neighbor who told her Pastor about our situation and he was able to get a lead on a rental home. I had never had a washer and dryer before and a friend traded me a stove I had for a W&D. This was the middle of Dec. and people from that same Church donated money and bless their hearts and others, my kids had a better Christmas than they had ever had.

I fell down a full flight of stairs and lost my baby due to the placenta ripping away. I didn't have Lupus but suffered from severe migraines that were debilitating. I didn't think I could be a single parent. But I did it. I had to go on assistance during this time and after losing my baby I went to college and began to work on a BSW degree. I didn't think I was smart enough. But I was.

I remarried a man who was everything my first husband was not. And Heather, I am a survivor. YOU ARE, TOO. You just don't know that, yet.

You will do all you need to do because you have three little people who need you to carry on for them. God promises He will not give you more than you can handle, so I am telling you the truth: You are stronger than you think and you, Heather, are a survivor. Every one of us Lupies believe in you and we are here to give you the encouragement you need. No one will expect you to run through this; it won't be easy, but when you take one step at a time, you will make it.

Now, I pray that God will bless you and keep you, dear Heather, that He will keep His hand upon you and give you peace IJN

Be well, my friend,
Val

Jessie's Story

Hiya, everyone,

So happy you are all here! I have to apologize, as I know this is really long. I really am initiating myself with a bang, lol. But to feel like any answers I get are well informed, I really want to tell all I can.

My name is Jessie, and I'm 33. Very happily married in Pennsylvania, USA, one living child, our daughter Payton who is 8 3/4 :-). I was officially diagnosed with Lupus last year, but I suspected and had tried to plead my case since 2005.

I had a successful pregnancy in 2000, but in hindsight I had some intrauterine growth restriction that no one ever detected, along with some diagnosed pre-eclampsia. Lupus and APS manifested in later pregnancies, resulting in three losses, one in each trimester of those pregnancies.

Other than that, I have had relatively tolerable daily symptoms, but have become more concerned as I have recently been sick and I am reading way too much info online for my worrying mind. I'm hoping some of you can alleviate my fears and at least shed some light and truth.

I have Lupus, Sjogren's, APS, Lupus anticoagulant (I think that's right), and I also have the marker that causes fetal heart block, don't remember is that's ro or la or something like that (although we did not knowingly experience this with my pregnancies) , and high ANA levels. I've had pleurisy a few times, a mono-type illness (never truly determined to be mono), and a blood clot in my leg last year. I have ALWAYS been achy in my joints and various unexplained pains, most recently in the last year or two an occasional heaviness in my arm that feels like edema, but is unexplained, so chalked up to Lupus.

I am on a low dose of Plaquenil, take warfarin for clot prevention, wellbutrin, hypertensive med, and a hypothryoid med. Recently acidopholus for thrush I developed after a small round of steroids (trying to force myself to eat yogurt too).

I got sick early last year in February, prior to my Lupus diagnosis, thought to maybe be mono and pleurisy. I had rapidly developed a fever of something like 103 in I'd say like two hours, and after a trip in an ambulance, the ER did NOTHING and I waited there for about another four hours with no treatment.

My husband took me home and gave me ibuprophen, and I slept the fever out for a few confused and tossing, turning hours. When a concerned doctor put me on a Quinolone because they weren't sure what was causing all this, I swear I was ready to bottom out.

I changed doctors and the new doc told me my liver was very "sick" (there's that word again), and put me on meds I no longer remember. I remember feeling really bad, and started to be afraid I wouldn't get better. They put me on a nebulizer with albuterol, and I think steroids.

Eventually I felt like I returned to MY normal. The day I started work again, I got into a bad car accident. Did PT for a few months and several months later developed a blood clot in my left leg. I think it was mostly below the knee, a small involvement above.

The doctor did not believe I had a clot, and told me it may be a baker's cyst, but nothing showed on the MRI or CAT scan. I pushed and pushed to do something else, this is NOT RIGHT, and I lost all faith in that doctor because he did NOT want to do any more but wait it out.

Lo and behold, a clot. I've come out of that basically unscathed, with a future of warfarin. Ugg. I changed doctors last year to one I think is pretty good. I'm mostly satisfied with him, got a great rheumy I am comfortable with, and I was feeling settled and like I could pay attention to the rest of my life outside of this stupid "sick."

I have now sorta developed a relaxed approach, like - okay, I have a name for all this crap I have gone through. Now I just need to take the pills and listen to my body, etc etc. No kidney involvement or major organ involvement that I know of, just the regular aches and pains, and the happenings of the last year with being what everyone else calls sick

BUT I got sick about five weeks ago with what seemed like a bad cold that just wouldn't let up. Two weeks or so into it, I finally relented and called my rheumy because it was starting to feel like pleurisy again. Rheumy is an hour away, so a quick visit is just not feasible. He prescribed a chest x-ray, and with the scan of what appeared to be clear lungs, prescribed a round of low dose steroids.

That didn't really do the trick, so I consulted my regular internal med doc at my rheumy's suggestion, and they threw me on a generic zithromax pack. Not much help. Felt better a few days into it, but went right back to where I was after day ten.

Med doc feels that I have bronchitis, pleurisy, inflamed lungs, possible infection. Now I am on a different antibiotic, amoxicillin, a 10 day 2x a day course, along with steroids. They want to avoid quinolones and sulfas for safety's sake.

Steroids are 40 mg for 3 days, and reduction of steroids by 10 mgs every 3rd day. Also nebulizer with albuterol; this definitely helps with the inflammation. I am so congested in my chest and it doesn't want to come out, I can feel the rattle in my lungs and some small wheezing, but I'm coughing less at night and feeling a bit better now. I'm on day 5 now, I think. I'm still getting so tired though, totally brain-fogged (more apparent brain fog lately), and it's definitely affected my ability to function like I want to. I tend to push myself until I can't anymore, and this is kicking my rear right now.

I asked my doctor if we were being aggressive enough because I'm worried, and he is sure this is the right course to take.

If you made it this far, thank you so much for reading!!!!!

I'm thinking - Couldn't this all be a flare and not just a simple, every day Joe Schmo infection? Can I overcome this? Should I be concerned about this being a downhill course I can't overcome?

I'm worried.

I don't like being sick, and I definitely HATE, HATE, HATE worrying everyone - I really don't like being "that person." But I'm starting to feel like I am.

Mostly I'm worried that I haven't taken this seriously enough. Could I die soon? I rationalize that I have no major organ involvement; I "just" sometimes get pleurisy. But now I'm scared.

Please, someone tell me I am panicking for no reason and I'm doing the right thing. I've read so much recently about "will Lupus kill me?" and the survival rate is 80% for 10 years after being diagnosed. I'm almost 2 years into that already. God...

I'm so sorry, I very sincerely hope this does not bring you all down. I am feeling poorly and I'm scared, and I really don't like these feelings, not that anybody does. I feel like I've been fortunate, but have I taken that fortune a little too cavalierly?

Thank you all so so much.

I really value your opinions,

Jessie

Tea Cup and Saucer

" When my daughter died, I turned on God with an anger I didn't know I was capable of. After, when I needed Him the most, I felt that I had destroyed my relationship with Him because of my anger.

Weeks later, I went to visit my best friend, Geri. She knew me good enough to know my very soul was bruised and a part of me died with my Suzy-Jo. She didn't hug me or come into my space. She sat across the room from me and listened and when I was spent and I had no more, she stood up and said, "You need a cup of tea in my best china teacup and saucer."

She offered no advice, no physical touch, and no shared tears...only a cup of tea in her best. In the midst of an ugly place in my life I drank the tea from a vessel of beauty. A simple act gave me a glimmer of hope and an opening to feel God's love once again.

And that, my dear Kim, is the reason for asking you to do what I suggested when you felt it was too hard to keep going on. You are a vessel of beauty.

Be well

Val

PS: If you do not have a pretty cup and saucer I will mail you one of mine.

Frustrated & Depressed About 1st Rheumy Appointment

Robyn,

Welcome to my world. Now, after thirty years of treatments for SLE, I have been told by the only Rheumy at our local Kaiser, that I do not have Lupus. Yeah, right.

I DO have Lupus Anticoagulant, I DO have TIA's due to Lupus, so how can I NOT have Lupus? Hmmmmm? I told this local idiot that he was too interested on patterning himself on Dr. House on TV. He got mad, but then he laughed and told me I was his most outspoken patient. Yeah, well, I don't fear doctors, I often don't think they have a brain on their stem.

So, honey, you can try Lupus treatments that are not life threatening, like Plaquenil (Hydroxychloroquine), which also can help with Rheumatoid Arthritis. I have taken it for years, but did stop it after the first five, just to see if it was really helping me. Boy, howdy, what a difference. It can take up to six months to fully kick in, but it is worth the wait if it can help.

Loving hugs,
MM

Trying to Get Blood Work/Labs From Doctor

"   I'm getting really ticked off because my rheumatologist isn't very responsive. I've left messages and the nurse doesn't call. Then I call back and get the nurse, but the nurse doesn't see blood work in my file. What's up with that? I've already had my appt with the doctor to go over them so they have to be there! I just want a copy of my blood work, but they say they won't give it to me.

So the lab (when I called them directly) said they don't give it out to patients and the doctor's office is slow as all get out getting back with me.

Why is it that I can PAY for the labs, but no one will be helpful to give me a copy? They have laws about who they can share their information with, but won't give the actual patient the information? ??

I'm sorry to rant.... the rheumotologist's office said they'd fax to my family physician so I asked them to do that. I called the family physician and they don't have it. I want my lab work to get a 2nd opinion. What do I do now?

Vickie

Lupus and Diabetes

I was wrongly dx'ed as a T2 Diabetic (I turned out to be neither T1 or T2, but a rare AUTOIMMUNE T1 &1/2, yrs later) I had awful reactions to most of the oral drugs and none helped control my blood sugars. I told my doctors, one a GP who side specialized in Diabetes care (5 yrs) and one Endocrinologist (3yrs), that I felt AWFUL when on them, like I was being poisoned...both dismissed that as nonsense and both blamed me for 'non compliance'.

I went thru ALL the orals and various combo's of the orals, being sicker and sicker until I was about dead, working when I was dx'ed but was now confined to my bed (my son was 5) and DYING!

Only by GOD's grace was I able to somehow...get out of my deathbed, and started researching the Internet (I was computer illiterate to start!) and found research talking about this rare Diabetes, if you met 3 of their 5 criteria, you had it. I met ALL 5, no surprise to me! I fired those Dr's, went on 2 different Insulins, and 2 yrs ago WAS dx'ed as Lupus...that Diabetes had been one of my major symptoms.

Most of the orals are SULFA based, and so I was being poisoned and the orals NEVER work on this type of Diabetes, only Insulins! Never give up, listen to your bodies, it IS NOT in your head, FIRE any Doctor who suggests or tells you that (then fire AT that one!) Let's all pray for more good, caring, and curious Doctors.

GOD bless them...and all of us with Autoimmune Diseases.

. Amen!
Texas Carol

"Well; I'm stumped! We'll have to wait for the autopsy."

Found unattached to any messages.....Love it!

Lighting and Lupus

When I first got dx'ed in May 3007, my rheumy told me under ADA your work must accommodate the lighting w/appropriate filters for fluorescent lighting & these new bulbs are now everywhere. How come no one has done anything to make sure we are accommodated in every public place? I've been hollering about this to my friend's & family, but this truly needs to be tackled worldwide by the ADA!

Naomi

From the Archives: Summer 2009 Issue of Lupus Now

Lighting the Way
by Emily Wojcik

If you have Lupus, chances are you're familiar with photosensitivity, or abnormal sensitivity to light. Between 40 and 70 percent of people with systemic Lupus find their disease is made worse by exposure to ultraviolet (UV) rays, and the lesions of cutaneous Lupus are highly photosensitive. The sun is the major source of ultraviolet light, but UV rays also come from indoor lighting, like energy-efficient compact fluorescent light bulbs. Since the Energy Independence and Security Act was enacted in December 2007 -- requiring that all light bulbs in the United States use 30 percent less energy by 2012 and 70 percent less by 2020 -- these bulbs have become a hot trend. But what sort of risk do they pose for people with Lupus?

OMG!!! I am soooooo glad someone has finally addressed this issue. I have been dealing with this problem at my job, along with the glare these lights put out. Most every day I leave my work place with my eyes burning, red & so tired that I've had to take a cat nap before I can even walk to my car to leave. My boss thinks I'm nuts & making this stuff up, so nothing is being done to help me with this problem. That's a factory job for you. So therefore I have started wearing my sunscreen at work, covering all my exposed skin, including my eyes. Which for the most part has helped, & re-applying as needed. I have also started wearing tinted glasses too.

Thanks so much put putting this information out, so now I don't feel like I'm going crazy

Naomi

Neck and Facial Swelling

I occasionally got a swollen eyelid that looked like someone punched me, minus the black and blue. Came out of nowhere and nothing I did got rid of it. Happens for no apparent reason, but I suspect it is linked to a flare or low-lying flare.

Jessie

Lupus and Ménière's

My FIL has Meniere's Disease and has quite an awful time of it. He can't ride in cars for anything other than a very short trip and if he needs to travel usually takes the train. He lives 2hrs drive away but when he comes to visit he takes a 5hr train ride instead because he can't handle a long journey in the car. If he turns his head too fast he says he still has the image in his mind of what he was looking at rather than what he is looking at. He now has to walk around with a cane because of it.

A week or two ago I had a couple of days of dizziness which I imagine was mild compared to what he experiences but it gave me a new understanding of what it must be like!

Previously I have only had the odd episode where I would lose sense of the right way up, particularly if I have been pushing myself too hard. It would be a single episode however, and once I righted myself I was ok. I haven't fallen over yet. I basically just sat down as much as I could when I had the two days of dizziness to avoid falling over.

Is it a common symptom to have dizzy episodes?

Robyn Gough

Death in the Family

After her 30-year battle with Lupus and a fight worthy of being called CHAMPION,
my momma is tired and her poor body just cannot take anymore

suffering. We have decided "with mommas blessing" to let her go. It is the hardest thing I have ever had to do by far. She will enter into comfort care tomorrow afternoon. She will be given a constant morphine drip and will be taken from the machines sustaining her life. She will be allowed to pass peacefully and uninterrupted to at last be free of her broken body and pain that she has come to know so well.

She received her Last Rights tonight and is now in God's hands. Momma has been on life support off and on since January 1st of this year with a total of 37 days out of the hospital in all.

It is time. She is tired and she agrees. For those of you who have been through this before, I commend you on your strength because I just don't know if I can hold it together. I don't know how to do this without in some way feeling responsible for the outcome. I know no sleep or peace right now and I pray it comes quickly. Please pray "for those who pray" or send good thoughts, wishes for a peaceful passing and for those of us falling apart at the seams to find peace in this painfully confusing time. Thank you all, for being here for me. I have no one else to turn to, so you are my surrogate family in this time and I thank you for that.

Blessings,
Heidi

Update:

I know it has been a long time since I last posted (21 days to be exact) which was the day we took Momma off life support. She suffered for 19 long days. Up to 54 mg. of Dilaudid per hour, 400 mg. Fentanyl patches and 5 mg. pushes of Adivan every 15 minutes and still in pain. Thank God it is over and she is in peace. No one should suffer in that way. I ordered purple (Someone you know has Lupus) bracelets from the LFA to hand out at her service this Saturday

We've got to get this awful disease the attention it deserves. I have vowed to change my health in every way possible from today on. I refuse to let it get me the way it got Momma.

I WILL bring awareness to all who do not know...For me, for you and for my children. I will FIGHT THIS!

Blessings,
Heidi

What? Another Change in Diagnosis? Really?

Teri,

Doctors...the little dears. NOT. Honey, there is no definitive test for Lupus. There are many indicators, eleven of which are the most recognizable. The general rule is if you have four of the major indicators, you have Lupus. I have nine of the damn things, but my ANA titers are all over the map, so after thirty years of Plaquenil, NSAIDS, and other types of autoimmune drugs, the ONE rheumy at our local Kaiser facility says "You do not have Lupus." What a Moroon, to quote the great Bugs Bunny.

I have had some of the best doctors on the west coast, including UCSF Medical Center confirm the SLE dx, but this idiot thinks he knows it all from one blood test. My first rule of thumb is, "Believe what your body is telling you...not necessarily what the doctor says."

Find another Rheumy, or get your current one to shut up and listen to you.

Loving hugs,
MM

Pain Management

I was told today that Lupus patients DO NOT HAVE PAIN.

What idiot told you that? Pain was what got me to the doctor(s) and finally got a diagnosis. Today, I really don't have a whole lot of pain, thanks to taking Plaquenil for almost 22 years. Of course, I have pain from Fibromyalgia, and that's no fun, either. Today, it's manageable. But man, when I was in pain in the early stages of Lupus, I tried nearly everything and my doctors prescribed Imuran and Cytoxan and other drugs I can't remember.

The problem with someone else telling you that you don't have pain is that pain is subjective. You can't measure it scientifically, or see it, unless you are an astute person who sees a lupie doubled over in pain. Much of the time, we wonder ourselves if we are really experiencing "that much" pain. Well, how much IS "that much?" I, for one, was very stoic in my pain, telling only my doctors about it. And sometimes they didn't believe me, either, because "tests" don't show the degree of pain.

And I hate the old platitude, "I cried because I had no shoes, until I saw a man who had no feet."

Humph. When my feet hurt, my feet HURT.

Marilyn

Rheumy Upset Me

Angela,

Well, that doc visit sounds fairly typical of what we often run into. Nobody gets it, do they? These judgmental statements from doctors that we shouldn't blame Lupus for all our weird symptoms. My Lupus rashes and lesions not only itch like mad, but also can hurt for no apparent reason, and make my life miserable. I remember one doc telling me that the weird cysts I have had since early in my life were from not keeping clean enough. Daily showering, bathing, application of medication are not enough? What do I do, then, sit in a tub of water all day? The skin and internal cysts I grow are, according to UCSF Medical School caused by my body attacking itself. Well...duh. Hello, Lupus. Sheesh. Don't let it get to you sweetie. Research it, and then teach that idiot a thing or two.

Loving hugs,

MM

Loralee/ Re:Newbie Intro and Questions:

Loralee (pretty name),

Please always post anything that's bothering you because after being with this group for 3 years I can tell you honestly that you will ALWAYS get the very best advice, help, suggestions, etc from this wonderfully diverse and intelligent group of people. The only thing I would reiterate would be to stop yourself from doing too much research. It can really do a number on you and many times what you've read and understood to be what you're facing turns out to be something entirely different.

I speak from personal experience trying to get savvy about both my and hubby's health problems. You're just adding unnecessary stress to your already stressful life. I too am one who wants to have all the answers and have a full understanding of the situation so I can keep tabs on overworked, disinterested, incapable incompetent...or whatever... doctors; but just keep the research to a minimum. You know how you look the initial thing up and then it makes you think that it could be something else and then you look at the "something else" and you find something more.... round & round we go on the information merry go round till we're sure that we're not long for this world.

Take care
Georgia

Hello, and Thank You for Having This Group!

MM,

Thank you so much for your email! You definitely helped me put my mind at ease, it brought tears to my eyes to read and grasp your courage.

I wouldn't call myself courageous; yet, I guess a lot of my feelings are based on silent resignation to my current reality.

Losing our babies was such a terrible experience, one riddled with guilt and pain. I lived through it all, and it unbelievably brought my husband and me closer together. We learned about one another and how we really truly tick, bringing us to a better understanding of each other. I finally felt like I was coming out of our thunderstorm of loss, only to really start feeling the effects of Lupus as it decided to settle in. I so wanted to have a house full of kids, and I feel like my body cheated my family of growing. In this, I understand what you mean about feeling cheated.

I do consider myself fortunate, even with being scared and letting myself worry about my future. My husband is kind and soft with me, and loves me for WHO I am. He has been my rock, and has never made me feel guilty about anything (I don't know if I could be so strong if the roles were reversed). My daughter is loving and such a wonderful part of my life. A great student, someone I would have wanted to be friends with when I was young, so very witty and funny.

I'm not angry at my illness; I just want to do what will turn out to be right for me and my family. Your advice is something my best friend has tried to impress on me for so long. I am so used to pushing myself beyond my natural limits, I'm really not even sure what my limits are anymore. Has it caught up with me? Sigh... My past forced me to push myself (a long story), and I've continued that bad pattern in my present. I'm slowly learning now, I guess. I am having a hard time getting my husband to understand how drastically I feel I have changed in how much I can handle physically, and truthfully I can't blame him because I myself am not so sure until it's too late. Ugh...

You mentioned brain fog and nobody really understands what I feel like in that "fog." My memory and cognition used to be so sharp, but I can become confused for a second or two before I understand some things. Maybe that's just me getting older AND the Lupus, I don't know. I feel like I'm not 33, physically and mentally, but older, because of all I've been through so far. I hate that. I think I feel cheated in this way too, sad for myself that I can't get back the time I feel was wasted, or even time that was taken for granted.

I really have to get back to what makes me happy and helps me get centered. Feeling so vulnerable last night, writing my initial post, and now feeling a bit stronger reading your email and the email of others who responded...I think I have to listen to myself more, and maybe not be so selfless. I may need to learn how to say no and not feel guilty and anxious about saying no.

That will be a challenge. But I have slowly realized over the last 2 ½ years that I have really softened to others. I am a little slower to judge, a bit more understanding and accepting of people's individualities, and more respectful of those older than I. Maybe because I feel a bit closer to everyone, less self centered (is that a requirement of young adulthood? HA), so much more appreciative of what I have, we have, not coveting what we don't.

Thank you so much to everyone for being there when I needed you. MM, thank you for sharing yourself with me; I'm so glad you responded to me.

Jessie

Shingles Vaccine

I've had the shingles three times. They hurt worse before I finally break out. The last time I got them, I hurt so bad I thought I had broken my collarbone/shoulder. Then I saw the shingles rash. It spread clear up behind my right ear, and I still get some pain occasionally in that area.

I asked my doctor about the shingles vaccine, and he said definitely not. So we're all different, for sure.

Marilyn

Diagnosed?

I meant to reply to this and I think I got sidetracked... at least I hope I didn't already. lol Fibromyalgia is <u>perceived by the public</u> (and some medical practitioners that need to catch up), as being a "catch-all" label for a set of indefinable symptoms, but that is an erroneous view. Fibromyalgia IS a recognized diagnosis, and even accepted by disability as of last year I think it was. There have been changes in the name (Chronic Fatigue, Fibrositis) over the years, but it is clearly set apart now and found in any reputable medical book as such. It is a syndrome with a long list of conditions and symptoms. There are also clinical signs. The trigger points are only one thing. Fibromyalgia often presents with a low positive ANA, even in the absence of another disease such as Lupus (I didn't come up with that on my own, it's a statement from one of my Drs)

Tala

Lupus Editorial

Jesse,
What a great informative read about the fog.... loved it and read it to Mr. Carlson and he finally saw me as being normal.... sorta. Kudos.
I went to the PCP yesterday...sitting in his office waiting...eavesdropping on a conversation ...so much for confidentiality eh? just as he entered the room....I thought.... What the hey! Why am I here???

He sits down at the computer.... then looks at me and I am scrambling.... I had made the appt a week ago and for the life of me could not remember why...so I say to him, "Had lab work done yesterday and Neuts were 1.3 so I am thinking that the G-CFS needs to be upped to every 4 days. He does the hidden smile thing and says that sounds good...so I am thinking..."Oh and this is just likely a sciatic nerve thing but hurts like a son of a gun but not all the time...he said sounds like it let's see...did the muscle resistant thing...and then gets out the hammer and does the reflex stuff...he said sorry that may have hurt...I replied oh I didn't feel much as I have very little feeling in the feet from toes up to just before knee and on my hands up to below elbow...He sounds alarmed and says..., did this just start?.....I said.... heavens no, it has been going on for a long time now....he asked why I had not told him at previous appts and I said that I just thought it was part of the Reynauds and beside it didn't hurt so didn't worry about it.......his hidden smile is gone and he is just looking at me.....thinking.....obviously thinking......I said have you any input here as I have been self diagnosing and treating myself in your office.....when in fact I forgot why I was even here because I can't remember diddily squat anymore.......he looks at me and says......get this..........It is LIKELY LUPUS......go figure eh?......He says it is definitely not part of the Reynauds but would be neurological....which would make sense with the other markers I have. WELL BINGO! So the Rheumy says PROBABLE and now it is LIKELY.... who do I believe? Hehehe So.... like it always happens......... when I opened my computer last night and read your editorial it soothed my troubled mind... thank you for sharing with us.

Val

Shingles Vaccine

Hi everyone.

I discussed the shingles vaccine with my rheumy and he advised me to get it as long as I wasn't on any steroids at the time. I got it well over a year ago, as far into the week I could go to have most of my methotrexate out of my system. Of course I continued my Plaquenil and Cyclosporine. I also scheduled the vaccine just before I was scheduled for my Remicade infusion. I am happy to say that I had the vaccination and had to symptoms related to a live virus.

Everyone has to do what is best for themselves. Definitely discuss it with your
rheumy before getting it. It is now just one less thing I have to worry about.

Blessings,
Donna N/

Shingles Vaccine

Doc Said You Can Get Shingles Only One Time.... I Think He's Nuts....

Then I'm nuts, too.... I've had the shingles at least three times. Mine came from stress, I'm sure, since one outbreak occurred right after Christmas when I had the whole fam-damily for dinner.

Now when I hurt really bad along the neural pathway (behind my right ear, down to the neck, then the shoulder area) I look for the familiar blisters to show up.

Actually, it's a relief when I do see the blisters. Yep, your doctor would call me nuts.

And, I have residual pain along that pathway, too, sometimes. It's a gift that keeps on giving. Marilyn

Prednisone

Anita:

Have you asked her directly WHY she doesn't want to change or increase your meds? Sometimes you have to just be blunt and challenge the doctors who are keeping you from pain.... When my mother, who was 86 at the time, was experiencing horrendous pain due to her spine having spurs, etc. I went with her to her doctor's appointment. I asked her doctor, "Why can't you give her anything stronger for the pain?"

She answered, "I don't want her to become addicted to pain meds."

I answered, loudly, *"She's 86 years old. Let her become addicted!"* She got the pain meds. Plus some surgery later on.

My mother will be 91 next month and she's not addicted to pain meds.

Marilyn

Prednisone

Marilyn's right. Sometimes you just have to be blunt with them about the "why". They may want to be conservative, and that's admirable, but if something isn't working.... you need more or something else. It's ridiculous to stay with a treatment that isn't helping sufficiently (and unfortunately some Drs will if you don't get pushy about it). If there is a drug interaction she is concerned about, then she needs to explain it to you and offer you options. If it's not pleurisy, I'd say ok WHAT then? lol (You're not venting... and even if you were, that's allowed. I'd call it sharing. ;-))

There really are a lot of med choices out there. Sometimes they are reluctant for any number of reasons. The first one that seems to come up in their mind is drug-seeking behavior/addiction as Marilyn mentioned. It's ludicrous for most of us here, really. They are programmed to think that way, though. When you're asking for anything - not limited to a painkiller per se' - that should be the furthest thing from their mind. You obviously just want to feel better.

Tala

Kathleen DiSalvo's Story

When I was in my mid 20's I had some sort of strange issue with my eyes. They moved or what I called jittered all the time. I was nauseated and couldn't drive. Tests were done but nothing was conclusive. They doctor gave me tranquilizers and steroids and chocked it up to hysterical female! My next eye bout was a bit different. This occurred about 4 years later. I was in college and one day I woke up and looking out of my eyes was like looking at a curtain half drawn. Sort of like the roman shade being half up! I was a bit unnerved by this, naw I was downright freaked out! More tests were done and the only thing they could say was that it was a problem with my optic nerve. Steroids were again prescribed, which seemed to do the trick because my full vision came back.

During this time I also seemed to have issues with my leg dragging a bit and being very tired. Most of this I chalked up to being a college student with lots of stress plus I was "non" traditional because I was in my late 20's going to college for the first time.

I went to see a doctor at the Lubbock Health Science Center, he did more tests and said well we need to do a spinal and I said I didn't have the money, which I didn't so his best guess for all the eye issues, being tired and some of the other problems I had he diagnosed me with MS! This was a misdiagnosis.

Fast-forward about 8 years and I was out of college and working a full time job. In January of 1995 I started having lots of pain in my joints. Things were stressful at work and to make matters worse I hurt. On a scale of 1-10 about a 9 or 10 most days. It progressively got worse and worse. I was taking ibuprofen by the handful.

It all came to a head about March because I started running a fever and became bed ridden. I believe at its height it was a 104. I always said it fried my brain. Ha ha. Anyway at the time I lived alone and I called a friend to come help me. She freaked out and took me to the doctor. He said *oh you have the flu go home and drink plenty of liquids* and I think he gave me an antibiotic. In three more days I was worse and I am not sure how everything transpired but I ended up at the ER.

By this time I was in bad shape. I was severely dehydrated with a high fever. It took a nurse from Care Flight to get an IV started. At first they thought I might have bacterial meningitis. They did diagnose me with aseptic meningitis but they also did a Lupus panel. All the results came back with positive indicators that I had Lupus and aseptic meningitis. I was sick. My left lower lobe of my lung had collapsed, all the blood tests were off the charts and my sed rate was something like 50.

My friend asked me what she could get me and I said *a gun* because at that point I wanted to either be well or dead. The prolonged pain was enough to drive any sane person over the edge, but then add the other items and I felt it would be better to be dead.

After about 6 weeks I returned to work, but felt like crap every day. During the 6 weeks I saw a rheumatologist for the Lupus. He put me on a pretty high dose of steroids, which I stayed on for about 6 months. Slowly I got better.

During the months and years after that horrible bout I have had some minor issues. Most of what I am dealing with is minor. No major issues. My biggest problem was the secondary issue of Sjogren's syndrome. So I guess it goes back to my eyes doesn't it? As far as Lupus, I have to say I must be in remission or I was again misdiagnosed. I haven't been to a rheumatologist in several years.

And now, before I end this narrative, I feel I must once again, point out that although the majority of the messages and Lupus Stories are written by members of the Lupies Yahoo group, some are from other groups I was granted access to, but all of us who live with this illness will most certainly agree with the sentiments expressed in the message below.

Summing It All Up...

Hi, Fellow Lupies,

This is the third in a random series of writings from me to you on the subject of living Life in the Lupus Lane, and other aspects of coping with chronic illness. The Delete button is always handy if you get bored.

I was up extremely early this morning, around 5 a.m., sleep being elusive today, and I started thinking about how quiet and peaceful it is in our neighborhood at this hour. The only people out and about are the newspaper delivery cars, and the only noise their quiet motors and the "thunk!" as the paper hits the front walk. If I am super fortunate, it actually hits the front porch. That is a rarity. However, I have an early rising neighbor who usually puts my paper on the porch when he goes by while walking his dog. He also puts my garbage cans out for the collection company, and asks if there is anything I need done that my boys can't do for me.

Now, THAT'S what I call a good neighbor.

And, good neighbors are what I call all of you.

You take the time and trouble to help our fellow Lupies in their search for support, comfort, encouragement and knowledge, and are, in turn, comforted by them when you are in need of it. That's what good neighbors are all about...mutual support and caring. Every one of you has been a good neighbor to me and our fellow sufferers at one time or another, and I hope you feel that you can come to "the neighborhood" when you find yourself in need of caring support. We may not know exactly the right thing to say or do, but we are willing, eager to help, and trying our best, and that counts for more than just getting it right every time.

I remember, when I was young, a neighbor of ours lost a child to congenital heart problems, and that was in the days before such things as transplants and open-heart surgery. A beautiful little girl of ten, she had gone through multiple surgeries, treatments, and a long time at full bed rest, yet she was the most well-known and popular kid in the neighborhood. It was because she was always "there" to listen, read with friends, talk, and just sort of be with other kids, and that was a comfort and a gift to them. She was sorely missed when she passed away, by every child in that area. And, it was her laughter that was missed the most, I think. She found something funny to laugh at every day.

Such a wise person in such a young and sick body who found a way to make a genuine contribution to the world around her. She wasn't perfect by any stretch of the imagination and had temper tantrums, sad times, and unhappy times just like the rest of us, but she didn't have MORE than the rest of us in spite of her illness. I always thought she had a good excuse for being a spoiled little girl, but she wasn't. It took effort, I know, for her to be cheerful, and be there for the rest of us, but she did it, anyway. A truly good neighbor to us all.

I think that each one of you, in your own way, is like that little girl. You make a real difference to others because you make the effort and take the time to share. Whether it is to offer prayers, support, or cheering words, or to share your pain and sadness, it takes strength of character, effort, and perseverance to continue to do that in the face of the level of pain and fatigue that I know many of us experience on a daily basis.

You are open, honest, and caring people, and I commend you for being the good neighbors that you are. It is a privilege to know you.

Loving hugs,
MM, owner

Author's Note: I hope you have found some comfort in these messages, information, and compassion for those who have this devastating disease. If you would like to express your thanks, The Lupus Foundation of America would be grateful for any contribution you might give.

Information about Regional Chapters and how you may donate to our search for a cure is at The Lupus Foundation of America website.

I wish you good health.

Marilyn Celeste Morris
Fort Worth TX